Thermoacoustic Tomography

Principles and applications

IPEM–IOP Series in Physics and Engineering in Medicine and Biology

About the Series

Series in Physics and Engineering in Medicine and Biology will allow IPEM to enhance its mission to 'advance physics and engineering applied to medicine and biology for the public good.'

Focusing on key areas including, but not limited to:

- clinical engineering
- diagnostic radiology
- informatics and computing
- magnetic resonance imaging
- nuclear medicine
- physiological measurement
- radiation protection
- radiotherapy
- rehabilitation engineering
- ultrasound and non-ionising radiation.

A number of IPEM–IOP titles are published as part of the EUTEMPE Network Series for Medical Physics Experts.

Thermoacoustic Tomography

Principles and applications

Huabei Jiang
Department of Medical Engineering, USF Center for Advanced Biomedical Imaging, University of South Florida, Tampa, FL, USA

IOP Publishing, Bristol, UK

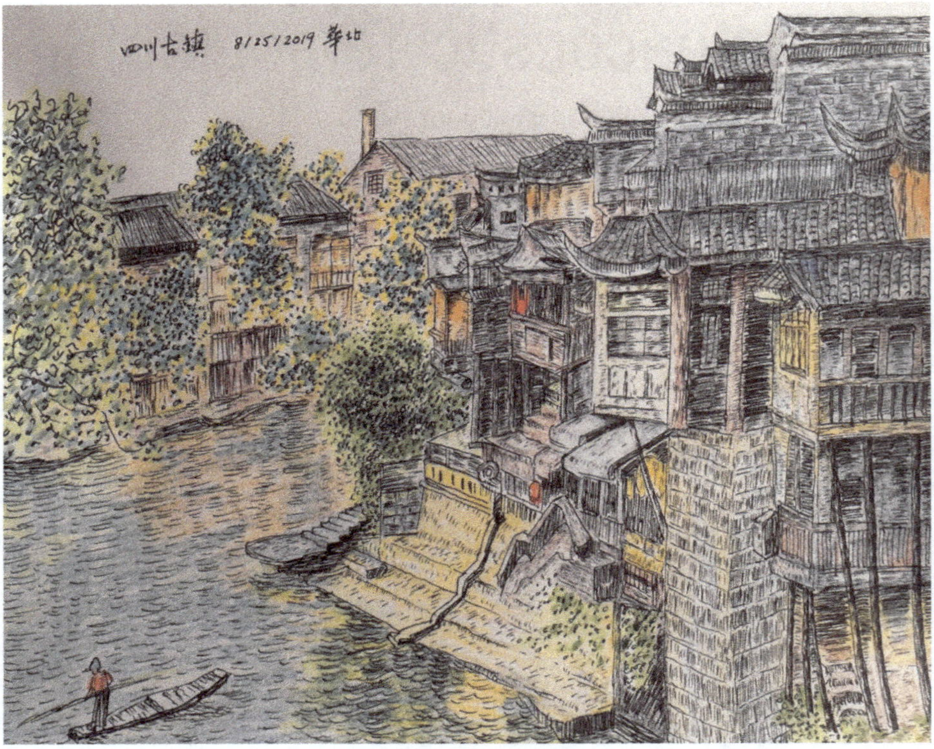

A historical small town in Sichuan, China. Ink and color pencil on paper, 27.9cm × 35.5cm, drawn and painted by Huabei Jiang. This piece was inspired by a unique combination of ink drawing and painting by impressionists.

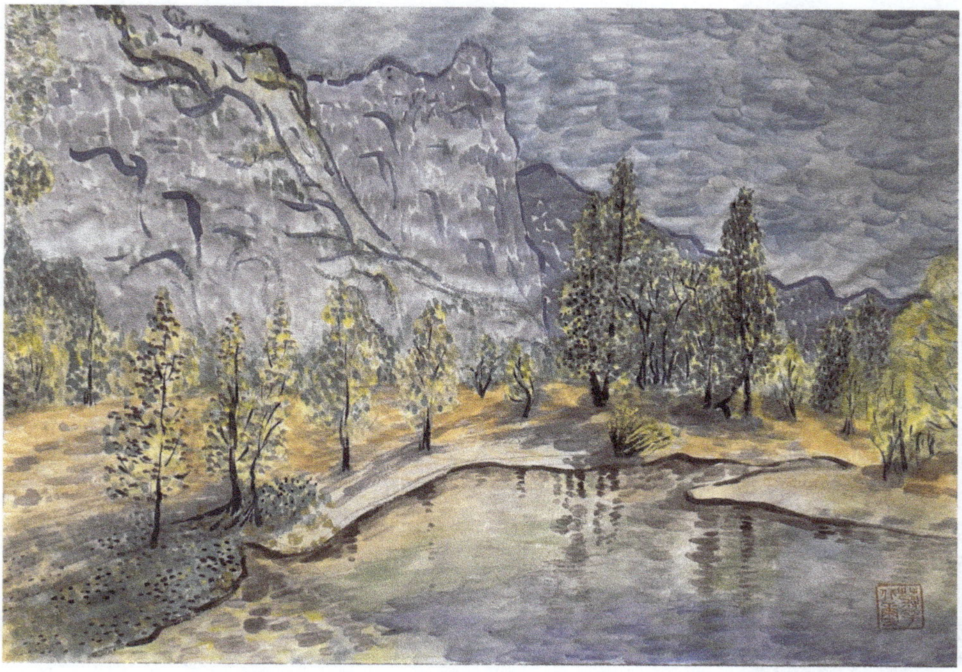

Yosemite National Park in California, USA. Watercolor on Xuan paper (from tree skins), 47.5cm × 69.5cm, painted by Huabei Jiang. In fact, this piece was inspired by conventional Chinese painting, watercolor and painting by impressionists, which is truly analogic to a multimodal approach in imaging science.

ISBN 978-0-7503-3163-0 (ebook)
ISBN 978-0-7503-3161-6 (print)
ISBN 978-0-7503-3164-7 (myPrint)
ISBN 978-0-7503-3162-3 (mobi)

DOI 10.1088/978-0-7503-3163-0

Version: 20200301

IOP ebooks

British Library Cataloguing-in-Publication Data: A catalogue record for this book is available from the British Library.

Published by IOP Publishing, wholly owned by The Institute of Physics, London

IOP Publishing, Temple Circus, Temple Way, Bristol, BS1 6HG, UK

US Office: IOP Publishing, Inc., 190 North Independence Mall West, Suite 601, Philadelphia, PA 19106, USA

To my Alma Mater high school, Quxian High School (Quxian, Sichuan, China), where I spent the most beautiful two years of my life.

Contents

Preface

Microwave-induced thermoacoustic tomography (TAT) is an emerging biomedical imaging modality that combines the high contrast and dielectric-based specificity of microwave imaging with the high spatial resolution of ultrasound imaging in a single modality. By listening to microwave, TAT detects tissue-absorbed microwave ultrasonically through the photo- or thermoacoustic effect. Since ultrasonic scattering is several orders of magnitude weaker than microwave scattering in tissue, TAT breaks the millimeters-scale spatial resolution limit associated with pure microwave imaging approaches for deep tissue imaging. In TAT, tissue is excited with a short (typically micro- or nanosecond levels) microwave pulse and the subsequent microwave-induced transient thermoacoustic waves in the range of kHz to MHz, due to the transient thermoelastic expansion of microwave-absorbing components in tissue, are detected by wideband unfocused or focused ultrasound transducer(s). Unique advantages of TAT are that functional parameters such as water content and ion concentration, and mechanical properties such as elasticity along with vasculature and blood volume can be imaged in high resolution. In addition, highly specific molecular TAT can be realized through the use of molecular contrast agents. Finally, TAT can be made portable for bedside applications, is economical, and uses non-ionization radiation.

TAT has found its potential clinical applications in several areas. In breast imaging, TAT offers submillimeter-resolution ability to quantitatively image the high microwave contrast generated through the presence of blood, water and lipid, which are the predominate transformations associated with malignancy. Application of TAT to joint imaging has been recently explored, offering an opportunity for early detection and monitoring of progressive diseases including osteoarthritis and rheumatoid arthritis. In this case, the microwave contrast is produced through the degraded articular cartilage, and the increased water content in the synovial cavity. Other clinical applications of TAT also start to appear, including vascular, liver and thyroid imaging.

While brain imaging and electrophysiology play a central role in neuroscience research and in the evaluation of neurological disorders, a single noninvasive modality that offers both high spatial and temporal resolution is currently not available. TAT may become such a neuroimaging modality both in animals and in humans. We show for the first time in this book (chapter 7) that TAT can noninvasively visualize brain vasculature and dynamics without the use of any contrast agent in adult brains. This opens a new way to detect and track neurological disorders such as stroke and epilepsy.

The concept of TAT emerged in the mid-1990s and the field of TAT is now rapidly moving forward. While there are several comprehensive reviews on TAT, there is no single book available yet. It appears timely to produce the first book in this field. This book is essentially a collection of the research work that the author and his colleagues have been pursuing over the past decade. This actually presents a unique feature of the book as it allows the principles of TAT and its applications to be treated in a systematic way. In addition, the collection covers almost every aspect on TAT from mathematics, image reconstruction methods, instrumentation, and phantom/animal experiments to clinical applications. I believe this book will be particularly useful for graduate students and researchers who wish to enter the field of TAT.

In chapter 1, the fundamentals of TAT are presented, including the theory on the photo-/thermo-acoustic effect, various image reconstruction methods, and instrumentation. Chapter 2 describes advanced methods for quantitative TAT, which allow the recovery of tissue conductivity and/or mechanical properties. Experimental validations of the reconstruction methods are also presented here. The development of several image enhancing schemes, including both software and hardware approaches, are discussed in chapter 3. Chapter 4 describes array-based TAT systems that are the foundation for the realization of 2D and 3D TAT. The recent development of high-resolution and multi-modality methods are presented in chapter 5. These works describe the nanosecond pulsed microwave excitation based high-resolution TAT, and the combinations of TAT with other imaging methods including ultrasound imaging (US) and photoacoustic tomography (PAT), which represent new directions in the field of TAT. Chapter 6 focuses on the discussion of contrast agents based molecular TAT. Chapter 7, the final chapter, describes the clinical applications and animal studies in the areas of brain, breast, joint, thyroid, liver and vascular imaging.

Huabei Jiang
Tampa, Florida
December 7, 2019

Acknowledgements

I wish to thank my previous and current graduate students/colleagues including Lin Huang, Zihui Chi, Zhu Zheng, Xue Wang, Yuan Zhao and Jinge Yang, whose contributions to the works presented have made this book possible. I would also like to thank the staff at IOP eBooks, especially the senior editor, Ashley Gasque who has worked diligently at bringing this book to fruition. Finally, there are my family, and dear friends/classmates, who made it all worthwhile.

Author biography

Huabei Jiang

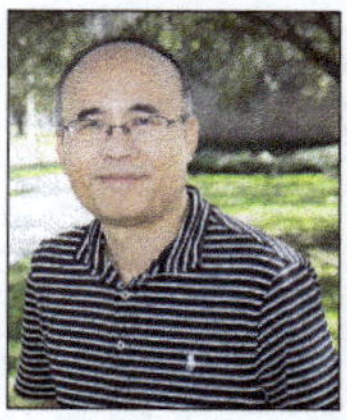

Huabei Jiang, PhD, started his career as an Assistant Professor of physics at Clemson University in 1997, and became a full Professor there in 2003. He then joined University of Florida (UF) in 2005 as a founding senior faculty member of the then newly established Biomedical Engineering Department and became the J. Crayton Pruitt Family endowed Professor in 2008 at UF. Dr Jiang joined University of South Florida (USF) in 2017 as a founding faculty member of the Medical Engineering Department and the founding Director of USF Center for Advanced Biomedical Imaging. Professor Jiang has published over 400 peer-reviewed scientific articles and patents. He is also the author of two books, *Diffuse Optical Tomography: Principles and Applications* (CRC Press, 2010) and *Photoacoustic Tomography* (CRC Press, 2014). Huabei Jiang is a Fellow of the Optical Society of America (OSA), a Fellow of the International Society of Optical Engineering (SPIE), and a Fellow of the American Institute of Medical and Biological Engineering (AIMBE). Outside his research/teaching, Huabei Jiang spends much of his time practicing Chinese Calligraphy and painting (ink/color pencil and watercolor), and occasionally writes poems in Chinese. He has had the first exhibition of his artworks in July 2019 in Chengdu, China.

Chapter 1

Fundamentals of thermoacoustic tomography

Microwave-induced thermoacoustic tomography (TAT) is based on the effect that acoustic pressure waves are induced in tissue whenever time-varying radiation is absorbed, which is considered an extension of the photoacoustic (PA) effect discovered by Alexander Graham Bell (1880), who observed that audible sound is produced when chopped sunlight is incident on optically absorbing materials. The concept of thermoacoustic imaging was initially conceived in 1981 (Bowen 1981); however, methods for tomographic thermoacoustic imaging or TAT did not appear until the late 1990s (Kruger *et al* 1999). TAT is basically concerned with an inverse problem where a single short-pulsed microwave beam illuminates an object and the thermoacoustic waves excited by thermoelastic expansion are measured using wideband ultrasound transducers in multiple locations around the object. The geometry of the object and spatial distribution of the microwave absorption are obtained from the measured ultrasonic waves using a reconstruction algorithm. In this chapter, we present the basic thermoacoustic wave theory, image reconstruction methods and essential hardware components needed for implementing a TAT system.

1.1 Thermoacoustic effect

Thermoacoustic (TA) wave generation and propagation in biological tissue is rigorously described by the Helmholtz-like wave equation. To derive the TA wave equation, three general elastic mechanical and fluid dynamic equations are responsible for the TA generation and propagation: Newton's law of motion, equation of continuity, and thermal elastic equation:

$$\rho(r)\frac{\partial}{\partial t}V(r, t) = -\nabla p(r, t) \tag{1.1}$$

$$\nabla \cdot V(r, t) = -\frac{1}{\rho(r)v_s^2(r)}\frac{\partial}{\partial t}p(r, t) + \beta\frac{\partial}{\partial t}T(r, t) \tag{1.2}$$

$$\rho(r)C_p\frac{\partial}{\partial t}T(r, t) = H(r, t) \tag{1.3}$$

where ρ is the mass density, V is the particle velocity, p is the pressure wave, v_s is the acoustic velocity, C_p is the specific heat capacity, β is the thermal coefficient of volume expansion, and H is the microwave excitation source term, i.e. the time-dependent locally absorbed microwave energy density. Considering equations (1.1)–(1.3) and eliminating V, we obtain

$$\rho(r)\nabla \cdot \left(\frac{1}{\rho(r)}\nabla p(r, t)\right) - \frac{1}{v_s^2(r)}\frac{\partial^2}{\partial t^2}p(r, t) = -\frac{\beta}{C_p}\frac{\partial}{\partial t}H(r, t) \tag{1.4}$$

If a homogeneous elastic medium is assumed, equation (1.4) is further written as,

$$\nabla^2 p(r, t) - \frac{1}{v_s^2(r)}\frac{\partial^2}{\partial t^2}p(r, t) = -\frac{\beta}{C_p}\frac{\partial}{\partial t}H(r, t) \tag{1.5}$$

Equation (1.5) is the general TA wave equation (without acoustic attenuation) in time domain. If a homogeneous acoustic medium is also assumed, equation (1.5) is written as

$$\nabla^2 p(r, t) - \frac{\partial^2}{v_0^2\partial t^2}p(r, t) = -\frac{\beta}{C_p}\frac{\partial}{\partial t}H(r, t) \tag{1.6}$$

where v_0 is the constant acoustic velocity within the entire problem domain.

Denoting the following Fourier transform expression for acoustic pressure,

$$P(r, \omega) = \int_{-\infty}^{+\infty} p(r, t)\exp(-i\omega t)dt \tag{1.7}$$

and taking the Fourier transform on equation (1.5) with respect to variable t, we obtain the TA wave equation in the frequency domain (assuming $H = \Psi I(t) = \Psi\delta(t - t_0)$, where Ψ is the locally absorbed microwave energy density, and $I(t)$ is the temporal illumination function—here a delta function is assumed):

$$\nabla^2 P(r, \omega) + k^2 P(r, \omega) = ik\, v_s\frac{\beta\Psi(r)}{C_p} \tag{1.8}$$

where P is the pressure wave in frequency domain; $k = \omega/v_s$ is the wave number described by the angular frequency, ω and the acoustic speed, v_s. The TA wave equation in frequency domain for a homogeneous acoustic medium is accordingly expressed as

$$\nabla^2 P(r, \omega) + k_0^2 P(r, \omega) = ik_0 v_0\frac{\beta\Psi(r)}{C_p} \tag{1.9}$$

where $k_0 = \omega/v_0$. If both the acoustic velocity and attenuation are heterogeneously distributed, the frequency-domain TA wave equation is then described as:

$$\nabla^2 P(r, \omega) + k_0^2(1 + O)P(r, \omega) = ik_0 v_0 \frac{\beta\Psi(r)}{C_p} \tag{1.10}$$

where O is a coefficient that depends on both acoustic velocity and attenuation as follows:

$$O = v_o^2/v_s^2 - 1 + iAv_0/k_0 v_s^2 \tag{1.11}$$

where v_0 is the constant acoustic velocity in a reference/coupling medium, and A is the acoustic attenuation coefficient.

1.2 Image reconstruction methods

1.2.1 Delay-and-sum beam forming algorithm

To form the tomographic TA image of an object, an image reconstruction algorithm is required. A simple, yet very effective method is the delay-and-sum beam forming algorithm that is commonly used in radar signal processing (Hoelen and de Mul 2000). The image expression in the case of near-field for thermoacoustic imaging can be stated as

$$S(r, t) = \frac{\sum_i w_i S_i(t + \delta_i)}{\sum_i w_i} \tag{1.12}$$

where $S(r, t)$ is the image output at a particular spatial point r within the imaging domain, $S_i(t)$ is the time-resolved acoustic signal from the ith receiver, δ_i is the delay applied to this signal, and w_i is an amplitude weighting factor, which is used to enhance the beam shape, to reduce sidelobe effects, or to minimize the noise level. Note that $\delta_i = | R_i - r |/v$ is just the time needed for the acoustic signal to travel from point r to point R_i, where R_i is the spatial location of the ith receiver and v is the assumed constant acoustic velocity. The summed signal is typically normalized to make the output independent of the actual set of transducers. This delay-and-sum algorithm has been tested and evaluated using considerable phantom and *in vivo* experiments (Huang *et al* 2017, Chi *et al* 2016, Ji *et al* 2012).

1.2.2 A-line/B-mode image formation method

The delay-and-sum method described above is usually used for TAT based on unfocused ultrasound transducer(s). If a focused transducer is used, its image can be simply formed by the A-line or B-mode image formation method used in conventional ultrasound imaging. In this method, one-dimensional depth-resolved images (i.e. A-line) at each transducer location are acquired and additional raster scanning of the transducer along a transverse direction (x or y plane) produces the 2D images referred to as B-scan. Further raster scanning along the other transverse direction enables the reconstruction of a 3D image. The thermoacoustic images can be displayed through cross sectional (B-scan) images, or maximum amplitude projection (MAP) images, where an MAP image is formed by projecting the maximum thermoacoustic amplitudes along a direction (typically z) to its orthogonal plane (x–y).

1.2.3 Iterative nonlinear algorithm

While the delay-and-sum algorithm and the A-line/B-mode image formation method described in sections 1.2.1 and 1.2.2 is simple to implement, they do not account for the diffraction effect that is essential to the TA waves. This limitation will certainly affect the accuracy in image reconstruction. In addition, acoustic and elastic properties cannot be recovered using these simple reconstruction methods. Most importantly, the TA image recovered using these two methods or other linear methods such as backprojection and filtered backprojection is not quantitative as tissue dielectric properties (e.g. conductivity) cannot be obtained with these linear methods (see more discussion about quantitative TAT in chapter 2).

To overcome the above-mentioned limitations associated with the delay-and-sum, A-line/B-mode and backprojection/filtered backprojection methods, here we describe a nonlinear reconstruction algorithm based on the finite-element (FE) solution to the full TA wave equation. The finite-element method (FEM) has been a powerful numerical method for solving the Helmholtz-type equation, because of its computational efficiency and unrivaled ability to accommodate tissue heterogeneity and geometrical irregularity as well as allow complex boundary conditions and source representations. This reconstruction approach in TAT is an iterative Newton method with combined Marquardt and Tikhonov regularizations that can provide stable inverse solutions. The approach uses the hybrid regularizations-based Newton method to update an initial microwave/electrical property distribution iteratively in order to minimize an object function composed of a weighted sum of the squared difference between computed and measured data. Together with the iterative Newton method, this nonlinear algorithm is able to precisely solve the Helmholtz wave equation and fulfill reliable inverse computation for an arbitrary measurement configuration. The nonlinear algorithm is implemented in both frequency- and time domain as follows.

1.2.3.1 Frequency-domain FE-based algorithm

The TA wave equation in frequency-domain is written if a homogeneous acoustic medium is considered (for the case of inhomogeneous acoustic medium, see chapter 2),

$$\nabla^2 P(r, \omega) + k_0^2 P(r, \omega) = ik_0 v_0 \frac{\beta \Psi(r)}{C_p} \tag{1.13}$$

Expanding acoustic pressure, P as the sum of coefficients multiplied by a set of basis functions, ψ_j: $P = \sum P_j \psi_j$, the FE discretization of the Helmholtz wave equation (1.13) can be expressed as

$$\sum_{j=1}^{N} P_j \left[\langle \nabla \psi_j \cdot \nabla \psi_i \rangle - \langle k_0^2 \psi_j \psi_i \rangle - \oint \left(\eta \psi_j + \gamma \frac{\partial^2 \psi_j}{\partial \varphi^2} \right) \psi_i ds \right] \tag{1.14}$$
$$= - \langle i k_0 v_0 \beta \Psi / C_P \psi_i \rangle$$

where the following second-order absorbing boundary conditions have been applied (Jiang *et al* 2006):

$$\nabla P \cdot \hat{n} = \eta P + \gamma \frac{\partial^2 P}{\partial \varphi^2} \tag{1.15}$$

where $\eta = (-ik_0 - 3/2\rho + i3/8k_0\rho^2)/(1 - i/k_0\rho)$ and $\gamma = (-i/2k_0\rho^2)/(1 - i/k_0\rho)$; N is the total number of nodes of the FE mesh, $<(\cdot)>$ indicates the integration over the problem domain and $\oint$ expresses the integration over the boundary. In both the forward and inverse calculations, the unknown Ψ needs to be separated into real (Ψ_R) and imaginary (Ψ_I) parts, both of which are expanded in a similar fashion to P as a sum of unknown parameters multiplied by a known spatially varying basis function. The matrix form of equation (1.14) is expressed as follows:

$$[A]\{P\} = \{B\} \tag{1.16}$$

where

$$A_{ij} = \langle \nabla \Psi_j \cdot \nabla \Psi_i \rangle - k_0^2 \langle \Psi_j \Psi_i \rangle - \oint \left(\eta \Psi_j + \gamma \frac{\partial^2 \Psi_j}{\partial \varphi^2} \right) \Psi_j ds \tag{1.17}$$

$$B_i = -I k_0 v_0 \beta \left\langle \sum_k \Psi_{R,k} \psi_k \psi_i \right\rangle \bigg/ C_p + k_0 v_0 \beta \left\langle \sum_l \Psi_{I,l} \psi_l \psi_i \right\rangle \bigg/ C_p \tag{1.18}$$

$$\{P\} = \{P_1, P_2, \cdots, P_N\}^T \tag{1.19}$$

To form an image from a presumably uniform initial guess of the microwave property distribution, we use iterative Newton's method to update Ψ_R and Ψ_I from their starting values. In this method, we Taylor expand P about an assumed (Ψ_R, Ψ_I) distribution, which is a perturbation away from some other distribution, ($\tilde{\Psi}_R$, $\tilde{\Psi}_I$), such that a discrete set of P values can be expressed as

$$P(\tilde{\Psi}_R, \tilde{\Psi}_I) = P(\Psi_R, \Psi_I) + \frac{\partial P}{\partial \Psi_R} \Delta \Psi_R + \frac{\partial P}{\partial \Psi_I} \Delta \Psi_I + \cdots \tag{1.20}$$

where $\Delta\Psi_R = \tilde{\Psi}_R - \Psi_R$, and $\Delta\Psi_I = \tilde{\Psi}_I - \Psi_I$. If the assumed microwave property distribution is close to the true profile, the left hand side of equation (1.20) can be considered as true data (observed or measured), and the relationship can be truncated to yield

$$\boldsymbol{J} \Delta \chi = \boldsymbol{P}^o - \boldsymbol{P}^c \tag{1.21}$$

where

$$\boldsymbol{J} = \begin{bmatrix} \partial P_1/\partial \Psi_{R,1} & \cdots & \partial P_1/\partial \Psi_{R,K} & \partial P_1/\partial \Psi_{I,1} & \cdots & \partial P_1/\partial \Psi_{I,L} \\ \partial P_2/\partial \Psi_{R,1} & \cdots & \partial P_2/\partial \Psi_{R,K} & \partial P_2/\partial \Psi_{I,1} & \cdots & \partial P_2/\partial \Psi_{I,L} \\ \vdots & \ddots & \vdots & \vdots & \ddots & \vdots \\ \partial P_M/\partial \Psi_{R,1} & \cdots & \partial P_M/\partial \Psi_{R,K} & \partial P_M/\partial \Psi_{I,1} & \cdots & \partial P_M/\partial \Psi_{I,L} \end{bmatrix} \tag{1.22}$$

$$\Delta \boldsymbol{\chi} = (\Delta \Psi_{R,1}, \Delta \Psi_{R,2}, \cdots, \Delta \Psi_{R,K}, \Delta \Psi_{I,1}, \Delta \Psi_{I,2}, \cdots, \Delta \Psi_{I,L})^T \tag{1.23}$$

$$\boldsymbol{P}^o = (P_1^o, P_2^o, \cdots, P_M^o)^T \tag{1.24}$$

$$\boldsymbol{P}^c = (P_1^c, P_2^c, \cdots, P_M^c)^T \tag{1.25}$$

and P_i^o and P_i^c are measured and calculated acoustic field data based on the assumed (Ψ_R, Ψ_I) distribution data for i = 1,2,...M boundary locations. $\Psi_{R,k}$(k = 1,2, ...,K) and $\Psi_{I,l}$(l = 1,2, ..., L) are the reconstruction parameters for the microwave property profile. In order to realize an invertible system of equations for $\Delta\boldsymbol{\chi}$, equation (1.21) is left multiplied by the transpose of $\boldsymbol{J}$ to produce

$$(\boldsymbol{J}^T\boldsymbol{J} + \lambda \boldsymbol{I})\Delta\boldsymbol{\chi} = \boldsymbol{J}^T(\boldsymbol{P}^o - \boldsymbol{P}^c) \tag{1.26}$$

where regularization schemes are invoked in order to stabilize the decomposition of $\boldsymbol{J}^T\boldsymbol{J}$; $\boldsymbol{I}$ is the identity matrix and λ is the regularization parameter determined by combined Marquardt and Tikhonov regularization schemes. It is found that when $\lambda = (\boldsymbol{P}^o - \boldsymbol{P}^c) \times \mathrm{trace}[\boldsymbol{J}^T\boldsymbol{J}]$, the reconstruction algorithm generates best results for TAT image reconstruction. The process now involves determining the calculated acoustic field data and Jacobian matrix. The reconstruction algorithm here uses the hybrid regularization-based Newton method to update an initial (guess) microwave property distribution iteratively via the solution of equations (1.16) and (1.26) so that an object function composed of a weighted sum of the squared difference between computed and measured acoustic pressures for all acoustic and microwave frequencies can be minimized.

1.2.3.2 Time-domain FE-based algorithm

The time-domain TA wave equation (1.6) for an acoustically homogeneous medium can be rewritten as (assuming $H = \Psi(r)I(t)$)

$$\nabla^2 p(\mathbf{r}, t) - \frac{1}{v_0^2}\frac{\partial^2 p(\mathbf{r}, t)}{\partial t^2} = -\frac{\beta\Psi(\mathbf{r})}{C_p}\frac{\partial I(t)}{\partial t} \tag{1.27}$$

where $I(t) = \delta(t - t_0)$ is typically assumed.

Expanding p as the sum of coefficients multiplied by a set of basis function ψ_j, $p = \sum \psi_j p_j$, the FE discretization of equation (1.27) is expressed as

$$\sum_{j=1}^{N} p_j \left[\int_S \nabla \psi_i \cdot \nabla \psi_j dS \right] + \sum_{j=1}^{N} \frac{\partial^2 p_j}{\partial^2 t} \left[\int_S \frac{1}{v_0^2} \psi_i \psi_j dS \right] - \oint_l \psi_i \nabla p \cdot \hat{n} dl \\ = \int_S \frac{\beta \Psi}{C_P} \frac{\partial I}{\partial t} \psi_i dS \tag{1.28}$$

The Bayliss–Turkel radiation boundary conditions are employed here (Jin 2002),

$$B_m p = 0 \tag{1.29}$$

where B_m is a sequence of linear differential operators,

$$B_m = \prod_{l=1}^{m} \left(\frac{1}{v_0} \frac{\partial}{\partial t} + \frac{\partial}{\partial r} + \frac{4l - 3}{2r} \right) \tag{1.30}$$

and B_m is subject to the accuracy,

$$B_m = O\left(\frac{1}{r^{2m+1+\frac{1}{2}}} \right) \tag{1.31}$$

This method provides an even more accurate approximation to the Sommerfeld radiation condition by annihilating higher order terms in $1/r$. However, the higher order (i.e. $m > 2$) boundary operators are not recommended for numerical implementation since they tend to spoil the sparsity of the FE matrix. As such, the first order absorbing boundary operator method is described as,

$$B_1 p = \frac{\partial p}{\partial r} + \frac{1}{v_0} \frac{\partial p}{\partial t} + \frac{p}{2r} = 0 \tag{1.32}$$

The boundary term based on equation (1.29) is rewritten as,

$$\nabla p \cdot \hat{n} = -\frac{1}{v_0} \frac{\partial p}{\partial t} - \frac{p}{2r}. \tag{1.33}$$

In both the forward and the inverse calculations, the unknown coefficients Ψ need to be expanded in a similar fashion to p as a sum of unknown parameters multiplied by a known spatially varying basis function. Thus, equation (1.28) can be expressed as the following matrix form in consideration of equation (1.33),

$$[K]\{p\} + [C]\{\dot{p}\} + [M]\{\ddot{p}\} = [B] \tag{1.34}$$

where the elements of the matrix are written,

$$K_{ij} = \int_S \nabla \psi_i \cdot \nabla \psi_j dS + \frac{1}{2r} \oint_l \psi_i \psi_j dl \tag{1.35}$$

$$C_{ij} = \frac{1}{v_0} \oint_l \psi_i \psi_j dl \tag{1.36}$$

$$M_{ij} = \frac{1}{v_0^2}\int_S \psi_i \psi_j dS \tag{1.37}$$

$$B_i = \frac{\beta}{C_p}\int_S \psi_i\left(\sum_k \psi_k \Psi_k\right)dS \cdot \frac{\partial I}{\partial t} \tag{1.38}$$

$$\{p\} = \{p_1, p_2, \cdots p_N\}^T \tag{1.39}$$

$$\{\dot{p}\} = \left\{\frac{\partial p_1}{\partial t}, \frac{\partial p_2}{\partial t}, \cdots \frac{\partial p_N}{\partial t}\right\}^T \tag{1.40}$$

$$\{\ddot{p}\} = \left\{\frac{\partial^2 p_1}{\partial^2 t}, \frac{\partial^2 p_2}{\partial^2 t}, \cdots \frac{\partial^2 p_N}{\partial^2 t}\right\}^T \tag{1.41}$$

Note that here Newmark's time-stepping scheme has been used for the discretization of time dimension (Smith and Griffiths 2004). The Newmark algorithm is a commonly used implicit method for the second-order propagation equations such as equation (1.34). In our case, we have

$$\{\dot{P}\}_{t+\Delta t} = \{\dot{P}\}_t + [(1-\delta)\{\ddot{P}\}_t + \delta\{\ddot{P}\}_{t+\Delta t}]\Delta t \tag{1.42}$$

$$\{P\}_{t+\Delta t} = \{P\}_t + \{\dot{P}\}_t\Delta t + \left[\left(\frac{1}{2} - \alpha\right)\{\ddot{P}\}_t + \alpha\{\ddot{P}\}_{t+\Delta t}\right]\Delta t^2 \tag{1.43}$$

where Δt is the time interval, α and δ are the time-stepping parameters which determine the accuracy and stability of the algorithm, $\{P\}_t$, $\{\dot{P}\}_t$, and $\{\ddot{P}\}_t$ are the values of the pressure and its derivatives at time t, and $\{P\}_{t+\Delta t}$, $\{\dot{P}\}_{t+\Delta t}$, and $\{\ddot{P}\}_{t+\Delta t}$ are the values of the pressure and its derivatives at the subsequent instant $t + \Delta t$.

Assuming that $[K]$, $[C]$, $[M]$, α, δ and Δt are constant, and from equations (1.34), (1.42) and (1.43), we obtain the following formula for calculating $\{P\}_{t+\Delta t}$ from $\{P\}_t$, $\{\dot{P}\}_t$, and $\{\ddot{P}\}_t$:

$$\begin{aligned}\left([K] + \frac{1}{\alpha\Delta t^2}[M] + \frac{\delta}{\alpha\Delta t}[C]\right)\{P\}_{t+\Delta t} &= [B]_{t+\Delta t} + [M]\left[\frac{1}{\alpha\Delta t^2}\{P\}_t + \frac{1}{\alpha\Delta t}\{\dot{P}\}_t\right.\\ &\left.+\left(\frac{1}{2\alpha} - 1\right)\{\ddot{P}\}_t\right] + [C]\left[\frac{\delta}{\alpha\Delta t}\{P\}_t + \left(\frac{\delta}{\alpha} - 1\right)\{\dot{P}\}_t + \left(\frac{\delta}{2\alpha} - 1\right)\Delta t\{\ddot{P}\}_t\right]\end{aligned} \tag{1.44}$$

The derivatives of the pressure at the subsequent instant are computed as follows.

$$\{\ddot{P}\}_{t+\Delta t} = \frac{1}{\alpha\Delta t^2}(\{P\}_{t+\Delta t} - \{P\}_t) - \frac{1}{\alpha\Delta t}\{\dot{P}\}_t - \left(\frac{1}{2\alpha} - 1\right)\{\ddot{P}\}_t \tag{1.45}$$

$$\{\dot{P}\}_{t+\Delta t} = \{\dot{P}\}_t + \Delta t(1-\delta)\{\ddot{P}\}_t + \delta\Delta t\{\ddot{P}\}_{t+\Delta t} \tag{1.46}$$

$\delta = 0.5$, and $\alpha = 0.25$ are typically used in the image reconstruction. When $\delta \geqslant 0.5$, and $\alpha \geqslant 0.25(0.5 + \delta)^2$, the Newmark algorithm preserves unconditional stability, which means that the amount of Δt does not affect the stability of the solution to the equation (Bath 1976).

Following the procedures described in section 1.2.3.1, the matrix equation for inversion can be written as

$$(J_t^T J_t + \lambda I)\Delta\chi = J_t^T(P_t^o - P_t^c) \tag{1.47}$$

where J_t is the time-dependent Jacobian matrix formed by $\frac{\partial P}{\partial \Psi}$ at each time step, $P_t^{o,c}$ is the time-dependent measured and calculated acoustic field data for $i = 1, 2, \cdots M$ boundary locations, $\Delta\chi = (\Delta\Psi_1, \Delta\Psi_2, \cdots \Delta\Psi_N)^T$ is the updating vector, I is the identity matrix and λ is the regularization parameter determined by combined Marquardt and Tikhonov regularization schemes. Here the submatrix of the Jacobian for each time step is assembled to form the full Jacobian matrix for all time steps. Thus we just need to solve equation (1.34) one time per iteration for the whole time range of interest.

1.3 Instrumentation

A typical TAT system consists of a short-pulsed microwave source (e.g. several microseconds), a single transducer scanning subsystem, and an acoustic signal detection subsystem (see figure 1.1). In this system, a pulsed microwave from a microwave generator (e.g. a magnetron at 3 GHz) is coupled into the sample via a coaxial waveguide switch coupled with a matching layer (for maximal microwave transmission) to generate an acoustic pressure wave. A transducer (1 MHz or higher central frequency) is used to receive the acoustic signals. The transducer and the sample are immersed in a tank filled with a microwave/acoustic coupling medium such as mineral oil or water. A rotary stage rotates the receiver relative to the center of the tank. One set of data is taken at multiple receiver positions (e.g. 180 positions) when the receiver is scanned circularly over 360°. The complex wavefield signal is first amplified by an amplifier. A data acquisition board converts it into a digital one

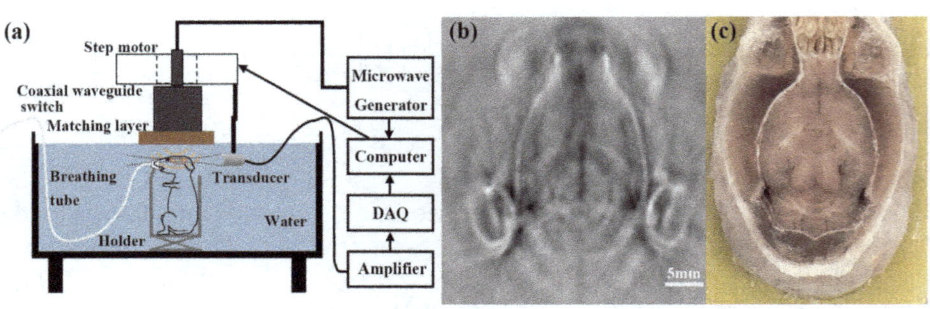

Figure 1.1. (a) Schematic of a typical TAT system. The sample here is a rat which is entirely immersed in water. A breathing tube is used to ensure proper breathing of the rat. (b) and (c) One slice of tomographic thermoacoustic image of the rate brain and photograph of the open-skull rat brain after the TAT imaging. DAQ: data acquisition.

which is fed to a computer. The entire data acquisition can be realized through C programming, for example. In this system, data collection for a total of 180 measurements may require up to 2 min.

In the typical TAT setup shown above, the mechanical scanning significantly reduces the speed of data acquisition. The use of a transducer array allows for considerably less data acquisition time compared to a mechanically scanned system, making real time data acquisition possible. In addition, a transducer array based system eliminates the use of water tank and allows the direct contact of the array with the skin (in this case ultrasound gel needs to be applied as coupling medium). The major drawback of an array based system, however, is its significantly added cost. We will detail an array based TAT system in chapter 4.

The microwave illumination pattern is typically an area—the key here is that the tissue needs to be illuminated homogeneously with sufficient microwave energy being absorbed. In addition to the circular scanning of a single transducer, or an arc or circular array of transducers, other types of transducer arrangements are possible. For example, reflection- or backward-mode microwave excitation/ultrasound detection can be realized, provided a compact microwave antenna is available. In such a configuration, the microwave excitation and ultrasound detection are performed at the same side, which is very convenient for applications such as thyroid and liver imaging (see chapter 7).

References

Bath K J 1976 *Numerical Methods in Finite Element Analysis* (Englewood Cliffs, NJ: Prentice Hall)

Bell A G 1880 On the production and reproduction of sound by light *Am. J. Sci.* **20** 305

Bowen T 1981 Radiation-induced thermoacoustic soft tissue imaging *Ultrasonics Symp.* (*July 1981*)

Chi Z, Zhao Y, Huang L, Zheng Z and Jiang H 2016 Thermoacoustic imaging of rabbit knee joints *Med. Phys.* **43** 6226–33

Hoelen C G A and de Mul F F M 2000 Image reconstruction for photo-acoustic scanning of tissue structures *Appl. Opt.* **39** 5872–83

Huang L, Li T and Jiang H 2017 Thermoacoustic imaging of hemorrhagic stroke: a feasibility study with a human skull *Med. Phys.* **44** 1494–9

Ji Z, Lou C, Yang S and Xing D 2012 Three-dimensional thermoacoustic imaging for early breast cancer detection *Med. Phys.* **39** 6738–44

Jiang H, Yuan Z and Gu X 2006 Spatially varying optical and acoustic property reconstruction using finite element-based photoacoustic tomography *J. Opt. Soc. Am.* A **23** 878–88

Jin J M 2002 *The Finite Element Method in Electromagnetics* (New York: Wiley)

Kruger R A, Reinecke D R and Kruge G A 1999 Thermoacoustic computed tomography–technical considerations *Med. Phys.* **26** 1832–7

Smith I M and Griffiths D V 2004 *Programming the Finite Element Method* 4th edn (Hoboken, NJ: Wiley)

Chapter 2

Quantitative thermoacoustic tomography

While the image reconstruction methods presented in chapter 1 and the linear algorithms such as backprojection and filtered backprojection seen in the literature can be used to provide high quality thermoacoustic images, the TA images provided are qualitative in nature as they represent only the distribution of absorbed microwave energy density or power loss density that is the product of the *intrinsic* tissue conductivity and the *extrinsic* square-amplitude of electric field within the irradiated tissue, indicating that the absorbed energy density as an imaging parameter of conventional TAT is clearly not an intrinsic property of tissue. It is well known that it is the tissue conductivity that directly correlates with tissue structural and functional information such as water content and hemoglobin concentration. Thus, a TAT method that can measure the true distribution of tissue dielectric properties will significantly extend the utilities/abilities of TAT, making possible high resolution quantitative physiological imaging of tissue at microwave frequencies.

While the term quantitative TAT primarily means the ability of recovering the tissue dielectric property distribution, we show in this chapter that quantitative TAT can also extract tissue acoustic property distribution such as acoustic velocity and/or attenuation, as well as tissue elasticity. It is clear that neither delay-and-sum method nor linear algorithms such as backprojection/filtered backprojection can do so. Fortunately, the iterative finite element (FE)-based nonlinear algorithms described in chapter 1 can be extended to achieve these quantification abilities. Here we describe thermoacoustic methods for recovering tissue conductivity, acoustic properties, and elasticity. Whenever possible, we use phantom or *ex vivo* experiments to demonstrate the validation of the quantitative methods.

2.1 Recovery of tissue conductivity

In this method, thermoacoustic measurements from the conventional TAT are combined with the electromagnetic Helmholtz equation to separate the product of

doi:10.1088/978-0-7503-3163-0ch2

the conductivity and the square-amplitude of electric field. Our reconstruction method for quantitative TAT includes two steps. The first step is to obtain the map of absorbed microwave energy density or power loss density, $s(\mathbf{r})$ based on the FE solution to the following thermoacoustic wave equation (considering equations (1.3) and (1.6)):

$$\nabla^2 p(\mathbf{r}, t) - \frac{1}{v_0^2}\frac{\partial^2}{\partial t^2}p(\mathbf{r}, t) = -\beta\rho\frac{\partial^2}{\partial t^2}T(\mathbf{r}, t) \tag{2.1}$$

where $p(\mathbf{r}, t)$ is the acoustic pressure at position r and time t, β is the volume expansion coefficient, $T(\mathbf{r}, t)$ is the temperature rise throughout the medium due to microwave absorption, ρ is the mass density and v_0 is the acoustic speed. This equation was derived from the equations of motion and thermal expansion assuming a homogeneous acoustic and thermal medium (see section 1.1).

Assuming microwave power dissipation in a region is so rapid that thermal diffusion can be neglected, the temperature rise in that region can be described as (Mashal *et al* 2009):

$$\Delta T = \frac{SAR \cdot \tau}{C_p} \tag{2.2}$$

where τ is the microwave pulse length, C_p is the specific heat and SAR is the specific absorption rate, defined as

$$SAR = \frac{\sigma\, |E(\mathbf{r}, t)|^2}{\rho} \tag{2.3}$$

where $E(\mathbf{r}, t)$ is the electric field, and σ is the electrical conductivity.

Note that the temperature transformation in the region is so rapid that

$$\frac{\partial T}{\partial t} \approx \frac{\Delta T}{\tau} \tag{2.4}$$

Thus, from equations (2.2)–(2.4), we can re-write equation (2.1) as follows

$$\nabla^2 p(\mathbf{r}, t) - \frac{1}{v_0^2}\frac{\partial^2}{\partial t^2}p(\mathbf{r}, t) = -\frac{\beta\sigma}{C_p}\frac{\partial}{\partial t}\,|E(\mathbf{r}, t)|^2 \tag{2.5}$$

If we define $E(\mathbf{r}, t) = E_z(\mathbf{r})J(t)$, where $E_z(\mathbf{r})$ denotes the spatial dependence of electric field and $J(t)$ denotes the microwave pulse function, equation (2.5) can be simplified as

$$\nabla^2 p(\mathbf{r}, t) - \frac{1}{v_0^2}\frac{\partial^2}{\partial t^2}p(\mathbf{r}, t) = -\frac{\beta}{C_p}s(\mathbf{r}) \cdot 2J(t)\frac{\partial J(t)}{\partial t} \tag{2.6}$$

where $s(\mathbf{r}) = \sigma \cdot |E_z(\mathbf{r})|^2$ is the power loss density and $J(t) = \delta(t - t_0)$ is assumed here.

The finite-element discretization of equation (2.6) can then be written as

$$\sum_{j=1}^{N} p_j\left[\int_S \nabla\psi_i \cdot \nabla\psi_j dS\right] + \sum_{j=1}^{N} \ddot{p}_j\left[\int_S \frac{1}{v_0^2}\psi_i\psi_j dS\right] - \oint_l \psi_i \nabla p \cdot \hat{n} dl = \int_S \frac{\beta s}{C_P} \cdot 2J\frac{\partial J}{\partial t}\psi_i dS \tag{2.7}$$

where $\psi_{i,j}$ is the basis function, and $\hat{n}$ is the unit normal vector.

The following absorbing boundary conditions are used (Bayliss and Turkel 1980, Mittra and Ramahi 1990):

$$\nabla p \cdot \hat{n} = -\frac{1}{v_0}\frac{\partial p}{\partial t} - \frac{p}{2r} \tag{2.8}$$

In both the forward and inverse calculations, the unknown coefficient $s(\mathbf{r})$ needs to be expanded in a similar fashion to p as a sum of unknown parameters multiplied by a known spatially varying basis function. Now the matrix form of equation (2.7) becomes available as

$$[K]\{p\} + [C]\{\dot{p}\} + [M]\{\ddot{p}\} = [B] \tag{2.9}$$

where

$$K_{ij} = \int_S \nabla\psi_i \cdot \nabla\psi_j dS + \frac{1}{2r}\oint_l \psi_i\psi_j dl$$

$$C_{ij} = \frac{1}{c}\oint_l \psi_i\psi_j dl$$

$$M_{ij} = \int_S \frac{1}{v_0^2}\psi_i\psi_j dS$$

$$B_i = \frac{\beta_e}{C_p}\int_S \psi_i\left(\sum_k \psi_k s_k\right) dS \cdot 2J\frac{\partial J}{\partial t}$$

$$\{p\} = \{p_1, p_2, \cdots p_N\}^T$$

$$\{\dot{p}\} = \{\dot{p}_1, \dot{p}_2, \cdots \dot{p}_N\}^T$$

$$\{\ddot{p}\} = \{\ddot{p}_1, \ddot{p}_2, \cdots \ddot{p}_N\}^T$$

Note that here Newmark's time-stepping scheme has been used for the discretization of time dimension (Smith and Griffiths 2004, Zienkiewicz *et al* 2005). The Newmark algorithm is a commonly used implicit method for the second-order propagation equations such as equation (2.9). In our case, we have

$$\{\dot{p}\}_{t+\Delta t} = \{\dot{p}\}_t + [(1-\delta)\{\ddot{p}\}_t + \delta\{\ddot{p}\}_{t+\Delta t}]\Delta t \tag{2.10}$$

$$\{p\}_{t+\Delta t} = \{p\}_t + \{\dot{p}\}_t\Delta t + \left[\left(\frac{1}{2} - \alpha\right)\{\ddot{p}\}_t + \alpha\{\ddot{p}\}_{t+\Delta t}\right]\Delta t^2 \tag{2.11}$$

where Δt is the time interval, α and δ are the time stepping parameters which determine the accuracy and stability of the algorithm, $\{p\}_t$, $\{\dot{p}\}_t$, $\{\ddot{p}\}_t$ are the values of the pressure and its derivatives at time t, and $\{p\}_{t+\Delta t}$, $\{\dot{p}\}_{t+\Delta t}$, $\{\ddot{p}\}_{t+\Delta t}$ are the values of the pressure and its derivatives at the subsequent instant $t + \Delta t$.

Assuming that $[K]$, $[C]$, $[M]$, α, δ and Δt are constant, and from equations (2.9)–(2.11), we obtain the following formula for calculating $\{p\}_{t+\Delta t}$ from $\{p\}_t$, $\{\dot{p}\}_t$, $\{\ddot{p}\}_t$:

$$\left([K] + \frac{1}{\alpha\Delta t^2}[M] + \frac{\delta}{\alpha\Delta t}[C]\right)\{p\}_{t+\Delta t}$$
$$= [B]_{t+\Delta t} + [M]\left[\frac{1}{\alpha\Delta t^2}\{p\}_t + \frac{1}{\alpha\Delta t}\{\dot{p}\}_t + \left(\frac{1}{2\alpha} - 1\right)\{\ddot{p}\}_t\right] \tag{2.12}$$
$$+ [C]\left[\frac{\delta}{\alpha\Delta t}\{p\}_t + \left(\frac{\delta}{\alpha} - 1\right)\{\dot{p}\}_t + \left(\frac{\delta}{2\alpha} - 1\right)\Delta t\{\ddot{p}\}_t\right]$$

The derivatives of the pressure at the subsequent instant are computed as follows:

$$\{\ddot{p}\}_{t+\Delta t} = \frac{1}{\alpha\Delta t^2}(\{p\}_{t+\Delta t} - \{p\}_t) - \frac{1}{\alpha\Delta t}\{\dot{p}\}_t - \left(\frac{1}{2\alpha} - 1\right)\{\ddot{p}\}_t \tag{2.13}$$

$$\{\dot{p}\}_{t+\Delta t} = \{\dot{p}\}_t + \Delta t(1 - \delta)\{\ddot{p}\}_t + \delta\Delta t\{\ddot{p}\}_{t+\Delta t} \tag{2.14}$$

The time stepping parameters are typically determined as $\delta = 0.5$, and $\alpha = 0.25$.

Following the inverse procedures described in section 1.2.3, the matrix equation for inversion can be written as

$$(J_t^T J_t + \lambda\mathbf{I})\Delta\chi = J_t^T(p_t^o - p_t^c) \tag{2.15}$$

where J_t is the time-dependent Jacobian matrix formed by $\frac{\partial p}{\partial s}$ at each time step, $p_t^{o,c}$ is the time-dependent measured and calculated acoustic fields for $i = 1, 2, \cdots M$ locations, $\Delta\chi = (\Delta s_1, \Delta s_2, \cdots \Delta s_N)^T$ is the updating vector, $\mathbf{I}$ is the identity matrix and λ is the regularization parameter determined by combined Marquardt and Tikhonov regularization schemes. Here the submatrix of the Jacobian for each time step is assembled to form the full Jacobian matrix for all time steps. Thus we just need to solve equation (2.15) one time per iteration for the whole time range of interest. The regularization parameter can be empirically determined, e.g. $\lambda = 0.8$ can be used in most cases.

The second step of our algorithm is to recover the electrical conductivity $\sigma(\mathbf{r})$ from the power loss density $s(\mathbf{r})$ obtained in the first step through a model-based finite element solution to the following scalar Helmholtz equation for electromagnetic (EM) waves

$$\nabla \cdot \left(\frac{1}{\mu_r}\nabla E_z\right) + k^2\varepsilon_r E_z = 0 \tag{2.16}$$

where E_z is the electric field, μ_r is the relative permeability, ε_r is the relative permittivity, and k is the wave number. While the detail on the solution based on finite element method for the second step can be found elsewhere (Ciocan and Jiang

2004), we give a brief outline here in order to couple the second step with the first step. The finite-element discretization of equation (2.16) can then be written as

$$\sum_{j=1}^{N} E_{zj}\left[\int_S\left(\frac{1}{\mu_r}\nabla\psi_i\cdot\nabla\psi_j - k^2\varepsilon_r\psi_i\psi_j\right)dS - \int_l\left(\frac{1}{\mu_r}\psi_j\frac{\partial\psi_i}{\partial n}\right)dl\right] = 0 \tag{2.17}$$

We use the second order Bayliss and Turkell radiation boundary conditions (Bayliss and Turkel 1980)

$$\frac{\partial E_z^s}{\partial\rho} = \alpha E_z^s + \beta\frac{\partial^2 E_z^s}{\partial\phi^2} \tag{2.18}$$

where α and β are two coefficients, and E_z^s is the scattered field:

$$E_z^s = E_z - E_z^{\text{inc}} \tag{2.19}$$

where E_z is the total field and E_z^{inc} is the incident field.

We can then obtain the matrix form of equation (2.17) which allows the solution of the electric field

$$[A]\{E_z\} = [B] \tag{2.20}$$

where

$$A_{ij} = \int_S\left(\frac{1}{\mu_r}\nabla\psi_i\cdot\nabla\psi_j - k^2\varepsilon_r\psi_i\psi_j\right)dS - \int_l\left(\alpha\psi_i\psi_j - \beta\frac{\partial\psi_i}{\partial\phi}\frac{\partial\psi_j}{\partial\phi}\right)\rho d\phi$$

$$B_j = \int_l\left[\frac{\partial E_z^{\text{inc}}}{\partial\rho} - \alpha E_z^{inc} - \beta\frac{\partial^2 E_z^{\text{inc}}}{\partial\phi^2}\right]\psi_i\rho d\phi$$

Thus we can determine the $\sigma(\mathbf{r})$ distribution by the following iterative solution procedure: (a) choose an initial value for σ, e.g. $\sigma = 0.0001$ S m^{-1}; (b) compute the scattered field E_z and its square-amplitude $|E_z|^2$ through the finite element solution to the scalar Helmholtz equation; (c) calculate the power loss density $s(\mathbf{r})$ by $s(\mathbf{r}) = \sigma(\mathbf{r})\cdot|E_z(\mathbf{r})|^2$; (d) compute the error between the measured S (from the first step) and calculated S^c, and σ is updated using $\sigma = s/|E_z|^2$; and (e) if the error is sufficiently small, then the iterative calculation stops; otherwise repeat steps (b)–(e) until a small error is reached. In the reconstruction, the incident field E_z^{inc} and the relative permittivity are estimated in advance. Thus, it is clear that unlike in conventional TAT, the microwave field distribution has been separated from the intrinsic tissue conductivity and is not part of the imaging parameter in TAT, which eliminates the impact of microwave diffraction.

Examples

Here we use numerical and experimental examples to illustrate the quantitative TAT image reconstruction approach described above.

In the simulations, the measured data were generated using a forward computation with the exact conductivity in place. A total of four cases having single or multiple targets were studied where the following known parameters were used: $\mu_r = 1.0$ H m^{-1}, $\varepsilon_0 = 8.854 \times 10^{-12}$ F m^{-1}, $\varepsilon_r' = 89.91$ F m^{-1}, and $f = 8.0 \times 10^9$ Hz. The 76 mm-diameter circular background had $\sigma = 0.1$ S m^{-1}. An area incident electromagnetic field was used for irradiating the entire surface of the background. A total of 120 acoustic receivers were equally distributed along the surface of the circular background region. The pulse width of microwave wave was chosen as 0.25 μs. The finite element mesh used for the inverse calculations had 1301 nodes and 2480 elements. All the images obtained from the simulated data are the results of 15 iterations from the image reconstruction (we found that a larger number of iterations changed the solutions only by less than 0.5%). Each iteration costs ~30 min on a 2.8 GHz Pentium 4 PC with 1 GB memory.

Figure 2.1 gives the reconstructed conductivity image for case 1 having a 20 mm-diameter single circular target with $\sigma = 0.2$ S m^{-1} where the exact conductivity

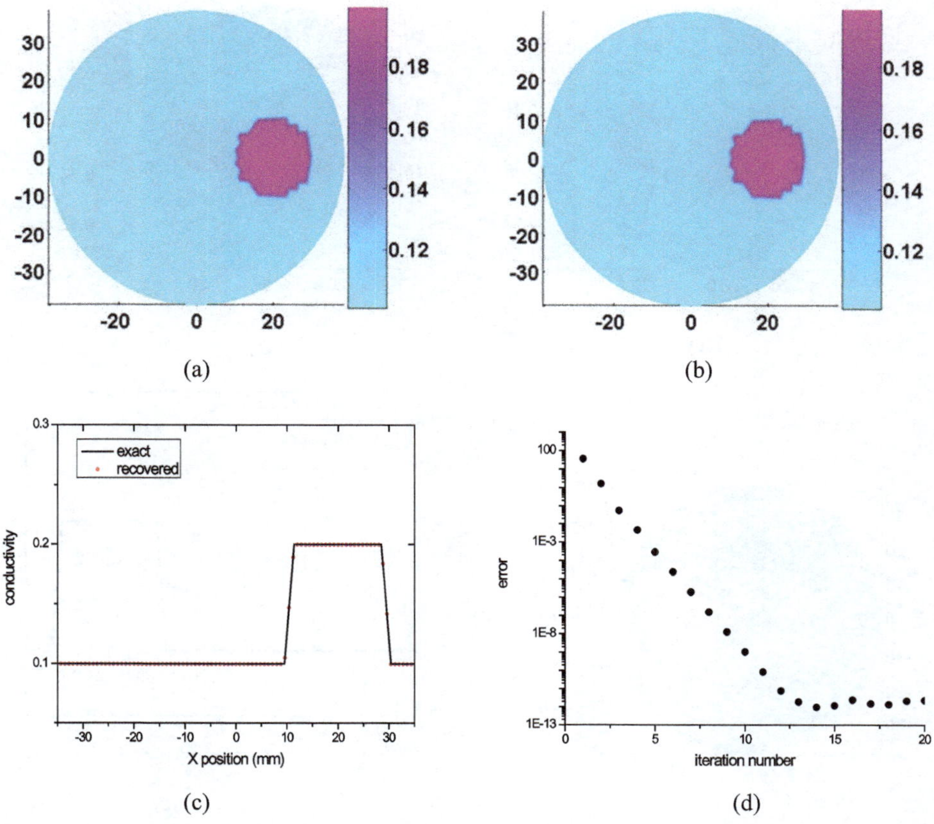

Figure 2.1. Reconstructed conductivity images for a single circular target without noise added (case 1). (a) Exact image, (b) recovered image, (c) the conductivity property profile along the transect $y = 0$ mm, (d) relative error versus iteration steps. Reproduced from Yao *et al* (2010) with permission, © 2010 John Wiley & Sons.

distribution is also shown for comparison (figure 2.1(a)). We see the recovered image (figure 2.1(b)) is almost identical to the exact one. The recovered conductivity property profiles plotted along the transect $y = 0$ mm, shown in figure 2.1(c), confirm the quantitative agreement between the reconstructed and exact conductivities. Figure 2.1(d) presents the relative error between the measured and calculated data over iterative steps in reconstruction where we can see that the error decreases rapidly and that the inversion process becomes stable after 12 iterations for this case.

Figures 2.2(a)–(c) provide the reconstructed conductivity images under the conditions of no noise, 5% noise and 10% noise added to the measured data for case 1. Figure 2.2(d) presents the quantitative conductivity property profiles along the transect $y = 0$ mm for the images shown in figures 2.2(a)–(c). As can be seen, our reconstruction algorithm is insensitive to the noise effect.

Figure 2.3 presents the reconstructed conductivity images for case 2 where the background contained three circular targets with different sizes (3, 6 and 9 mm in radius) having the same conductivity of 0.2 S m^{-1}. Figures 2.3(a)–(c) show the exact and the recovered conductivity images with 0% and 5% added noise, respectively,

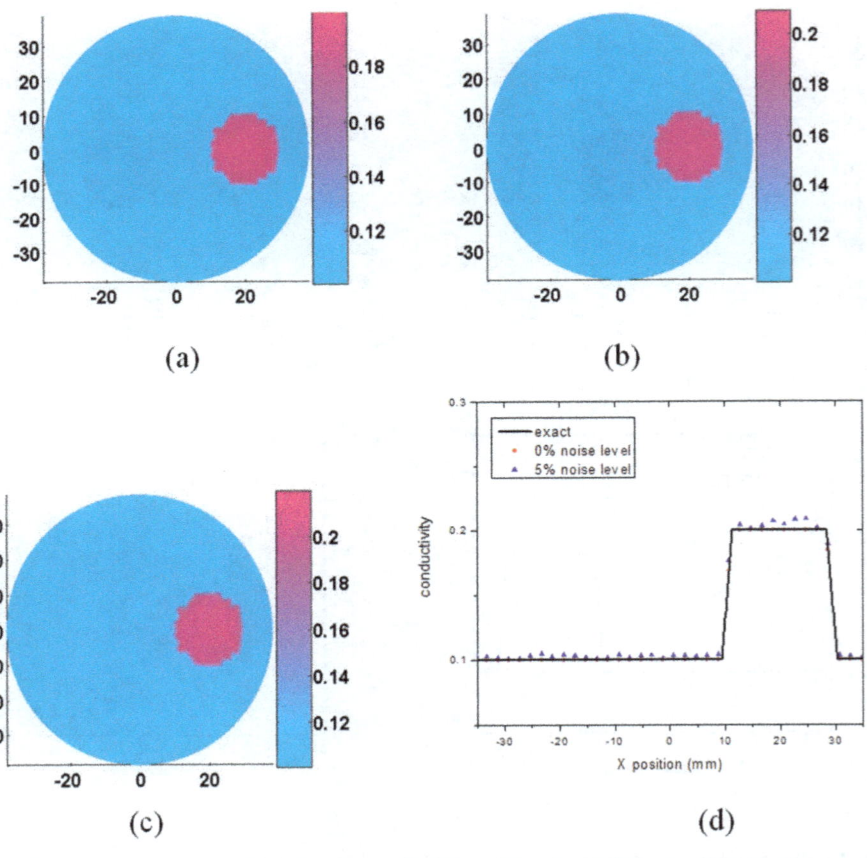

Figure 2.2. Reconstructed conductivity images for a single circular target with different noise levels (case 1). (a) 0% noise, (b) 5% noise, (c) 10% noise, (d) the conductivity property profiles along the transect $y = 0$ mm. Reproduced from Yao *et al* (2010) with permission, © 2010 John Wiley & Sons.

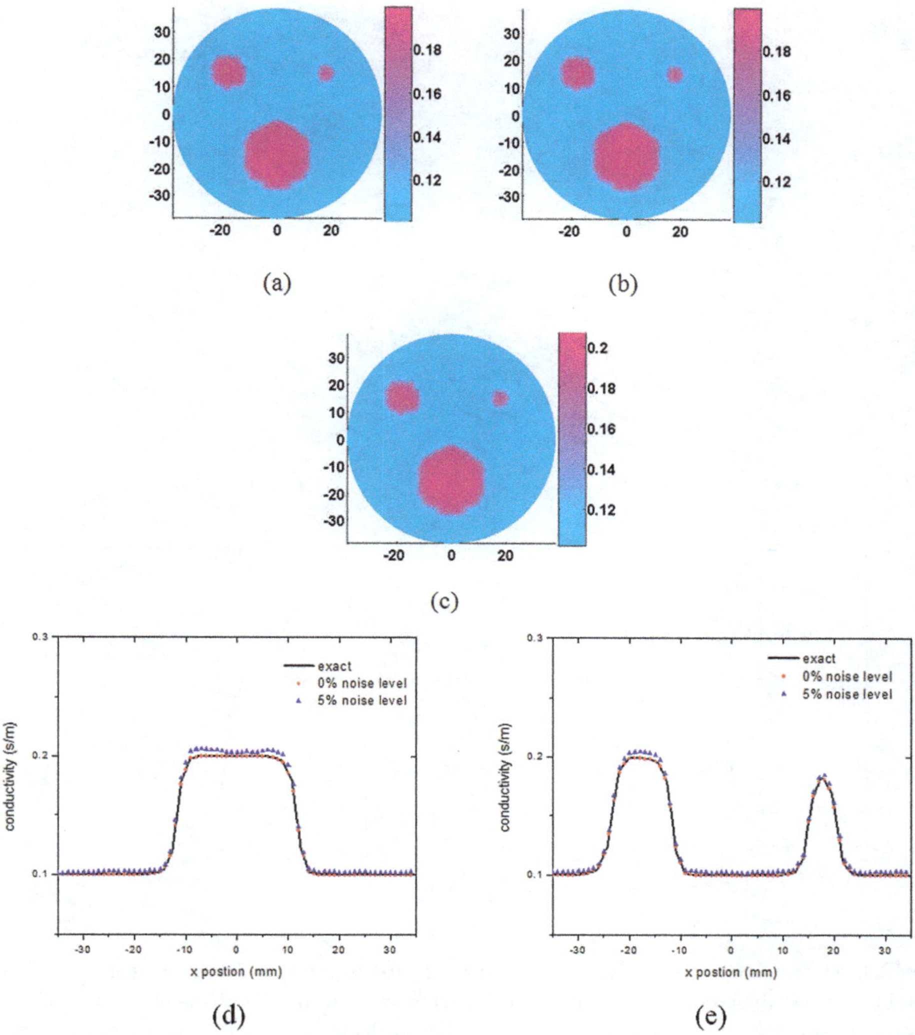

Figure 2.3. Reconstructed conductivity images for three circular targets having different sizes (case 2). (a) Exact image, (b) recovered image with 0% noise, (c) recovered image with 5% noise, (d) the conductivity property profiles along the transect $y = -15$ mm, (e) the conductivity property profiles along the transect $y = 15$ mm. Reproduced from Yao *et al* (2010) with permission, © 2010 John Wiley & Sons.

while figures 2.3(d) and (e) present quantitative conductivity property profiles along the transect $y = -15$ mm and $y = 15$ mm, respectively, for the images shown in figures 2.3(a)–(c). We immediately note that the recovered images are qualitatively and quantitatively correct in terms of the location, shape, size, and conductivity value of the targets.

In case 3 we attempted to test the ability of our algorithm for resolving different contrast levels. Here three 9 mm-radius targets having different contrast levels (0.2 S m^{-1}, 0.3 S m^{-1} and 0.4 S m^{-1}, respectively) were embedded in the background.

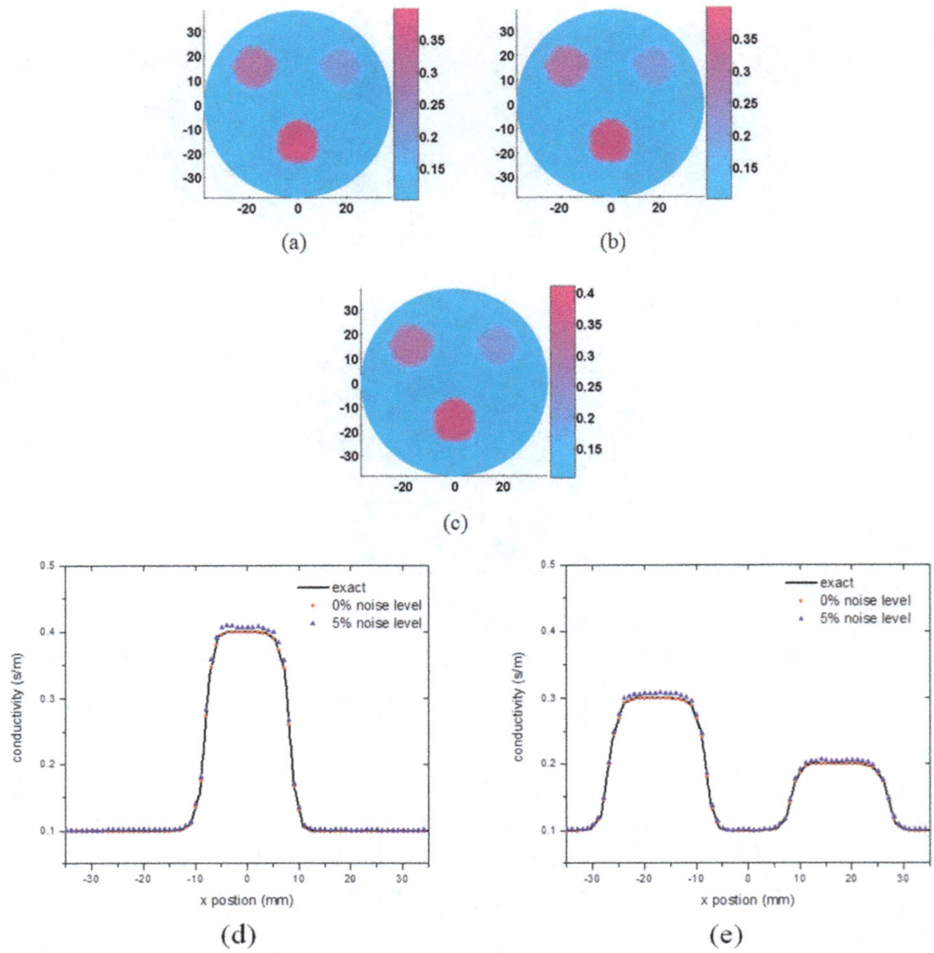

Figure 2.4. Reconstructed conductivity images for three circular targets having different contrast levels (case 3). (a) Exact image, (b) recovered image with 0% noise, (c) recovered image with 5% noise, (d) the conductivity property profiles along the transect $y = -15$ mm, (e) the conductivity property profiles along the transect $y = 15$ mm. Reproduced from Yao *et al* (2010) with permission, © 2010 John Wiley & Sons.

Figures 2.4(a)–(c) show the exact and the recovered conductivity images with 0% and 5% added noise, and figures 2.4(d) and (e) present the quantitative conductivity property profiles along the transect $y = -15$ mm and $y = 15$ mm, respectively, for the images shown in figures 2.4(a)–(c). These qualitative and quantitative results indicate that different contrast levels of the targets are clearly resolvable.

As a final example, we evaluated the ability of our method for differentiating three targets having different shapes (circular, elliptical and rectangular). In this case, the conductivity of these targets was $0.2\ \mathrm{S\ m^{-1}}$. Figures 2.5(a)–(e) show the exact and the recovered conductivity images as well as the quantitative conductivity property profiles along two transects. We see that these images are remarkably well recovered both qualitatively and quantitatively compared to the exact image (Adapted from Yao *et al* 2010).

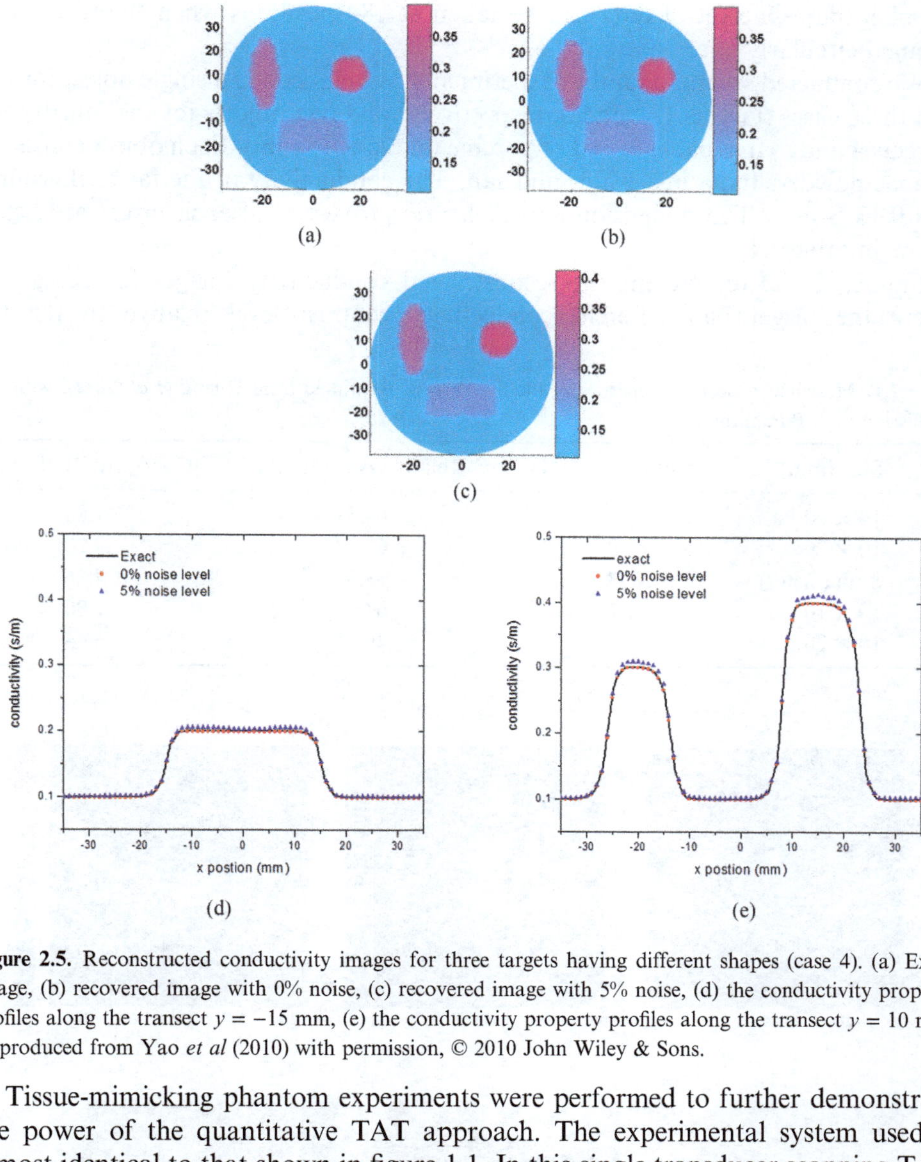

Figure 2.5. Reconstructed conductivity images for three targets having different shapes (case 4). (a) Exact image, (b) recovered image with 0% noise, (c) recovered image with 5% noise, (d) the conductivity property profiles along the transect $y = -15$ mm, (e) the conductivity property profiles along the transect $y = 10$ mm. Reproduced from Yao *et al* (2010) with permission, © 2010 John Wiley & Sons.

Tissue-mimicking phantom experiments were performed to further demonstrate the power of the quantitative TAT approach. The experimental system used is almost identical to that shown in figure 1.1. In this single transducer scanning TAT system, pulsed microwave from the microwave generator (frequency: 3.0 GHz, bandwidth: 200 MHz, peak power: 70~100 kW, pulse duration: 0.75 μs) is coupled into the phantom via a horn antenna (114×144 mm^2) to generate acoustic pressure wave. The actual microwave power at the phantom surface is less than 10 mW cm^{-2}, which is far below the safety standard (20 mW cm^{-2} at 3 GHz). A transducer with a central frequency of 2.25 MHz is used to receive the acoustic signals, which can provide a spatial resolution of ~0.5 mm. The transducer and the phantom are immersed in a tank filled with mineral oil for optimal microwave delivery and acoustic signal receiving. A rotary stage rotates the receiver relative to the center of the phantom. One set of data can be taken at 180 positions when the receiver is scanned circularly over 360°.

We conducted several phantom experiments. We embedded a single object for the first three cases (targets 1, 2 and 3, respectively) and two objects for the fourth case (targets 4 and 5) in a background of porcine fat (25 × 15 mm). Each object consisted of agar powder, India ink, water and salt. The conductivity of the fat background was 0.13 S m^{-1}. The dimension and dielectric properties of each target are listed below in table 2.1.

Figures 2.6(a)–(c) present the reconstructed conductivity images for cases 1–3 where the target had different conductivity contrast level relative to the fat

Table 2.1. Measured dielectric properties of the five targets. Reprinted from Huang *et al* (2012), with the permission of AIP Publishing.

	Size (mm)	Salt content (%)	Relative permittivity	Conductivity (S m^{-1})
1	10 × 20	1	64.37	1.80
2	10 × 20	2	61.34	3.20
3	8 (diameter)	3	58.34	4.36
4	10 × 10	1	64.37	1.80
5	10 × 20	7	46.55	6.44

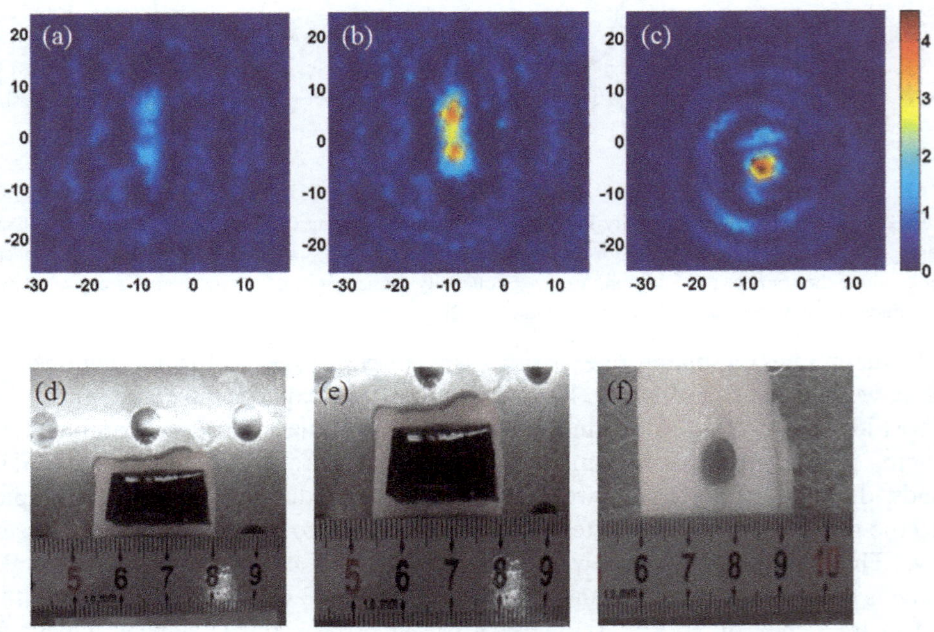

Figure 2.6. Reconstructed conductivity images for a single target having different conductivity contrast level relative to the background. (a) Case 1. (b) Case 2. (c) Case 3. The axes (left and bottom) give the spatial scale in millimeters, where the color bar (right) indicates the conductivity in S m^{-1}. (d), (e) and (f) Photographs of the phantom used for each case. Reprinted from Huang *et al* (2012), with the permission of AIP Publishing.

background. We see that the target in each case is clearly detected. In particular, the contrast level of each target is resolved. By estimating the full width at half maximum (FWHM) of the conductivity property profiles shown in figure 2.7, we found that the recovered object size ranged from 9.8 to 10.1 mm, which is in good agreement with the actual object size given in table 2.1. Moreover, the salt concentration used in our

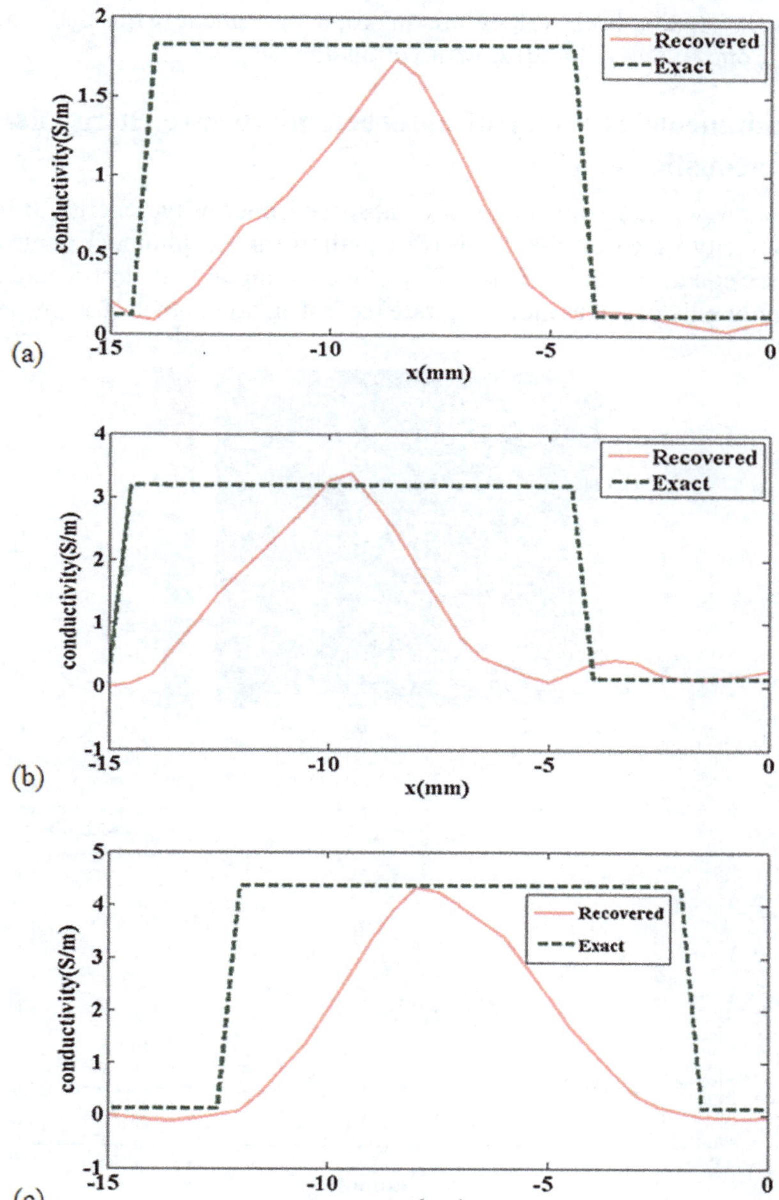

Figure 2.7. Recovered and exact conductivity profiles plotted along a cut line along $y = 5.5$ mm (a), $y = 5$ mm (b), $y = -5.2$ mm (c) from the images shown in figures 2.6(a)–(c). Reprinted from Huang *et al* (2012), with the permission of AIP Publishing.

experiments (1%, 2%, and 3%) gave a conductivity of the object of 1.80, 3.20, and 4.36 S m^{-1}, respectively. As can be seen from figure 2.7, we are able to obtain quantitatively resolved images in terms of the conductivity value of the objects.

The reconstructed conductivity image for case 4 is shown in figure 2.8(a). The recovered object size in this case was calculated to be 10.0 mm and the peak value of recovered conductivity is 1.92 S m^{-1} (target 4) and 5.93 S m^{-1} (target 5), as seen in figure 2.8(b). Again, both values are in good agreement with the exact ones. (Adapted from Huang *et al* 2012, with permission.)

2.2 Simultaneous recovery of absorbed microwave energy density and acoustic velocity

Here we show we can reconstruct both absorbed microwave energy density and acoustic velocity based on the TA wave equation for an inhomogeneous acoustic medium (see equation (1.10)). This ability of recovering both dielectric and acoustic properties not only provides more accurate reconstruction of dielectric property over

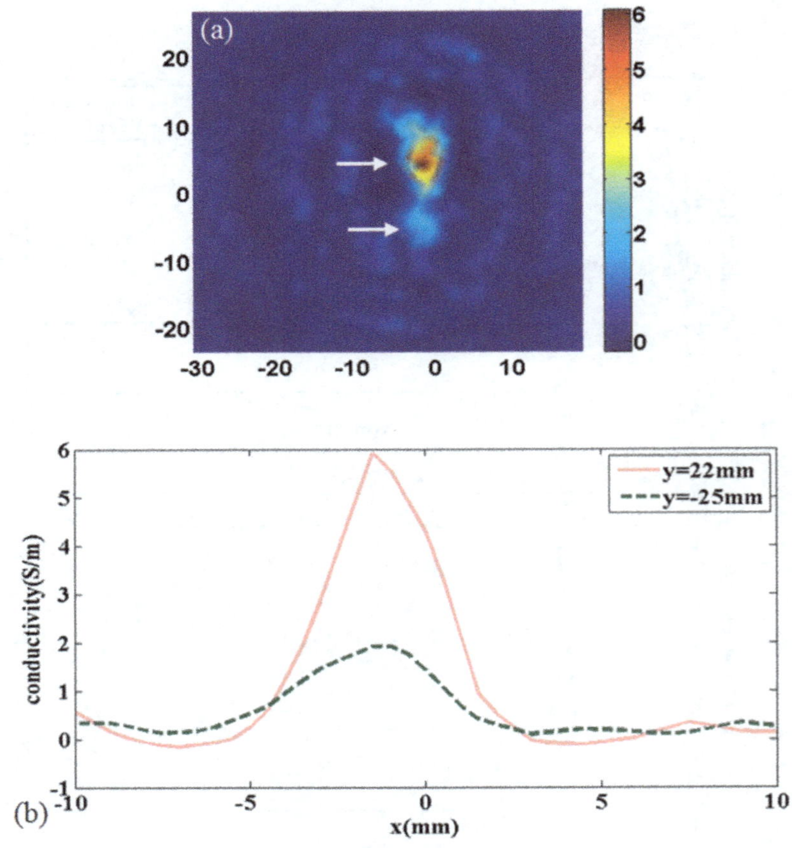

Figure 2.8. (a) Reconstructed conductivity image for case 4. (b) Conductivity profiles plotted along $y = -5$ mm and $y = 4.25$ mm from the image shown in (a). Reprinted from Huang *et al* (2012), with the permission of AIP Publishing.

the qualitative TAT because of the elimination of the assumption of homogenous acoustic velocity built in the qualitative TAT methods, but also adds the potential to better differentiate benign from malignant lesions as it is known that there exist significant differences in acoustic properties between normal and tumor tissues (Greenleaf and Bahn 1981)

The frequency-domain TA wave equation for an acoustically heterogeneous medium is rewritten here,

$$\nabla^2 p(r, \omega) + k_0^2(1 + O)p(r, \omega) = ik_0 \frac{v_0 \beta \Psi(r)}{C_p} \tag{2.21}$$

where O is a coefficient that depends on both acoustic speed and attenuation as follows (Jiang *et al* 2006):

$$O = \frac{c_o^2}{c^2} - 1 + \frac{i}{k_0}\frac{\alpha v_0}{v^2} \tag{2.22}$$

in which v is the speed of acoustic wave in the medium/tissue; α is the acoustic attenuation coefficient. The finite element discretization of equation (2.21) is stated as,

$$\boldsymbol{Ap} = \boldsymbol{B} \tag{2.23}$$

where the elements of the matrix $\boldsymbol{A}$ and $\boldsymbol{B}$ are expressed as

$$\begin{aligned} A_{ij} &= \left\langle \nabla\psi_j \cdot \nabla\psi_i \right\rangle - k_0^2\left\langle \psi_j\psi_i \right\rangle - k_0^2\left\langle \sum_k O_{R,k}\psi_k\psi_j\psi_i \right\rangle \\ &\quad - ik_0^2\left\langle \sum_l O_{I,l}\psi_l\psi_j\psi_i \right\rangle - \oint\left(\eta\psi_j + \gamma\frac{\partial^2\psi_j}{\partial\varphi^2} \right)\psi_i ds \\ B_i &= -ik_0\frac{v_0\beta}{C_p}\left\langle \sum_k \Psi_{R,k}\psi_k\psi_i \right\rangle + k_0\frac{v_0\beta}{C_p}\left\langle \sum_l \Psi_{I,l}\psi_l\psi_i \right\rangle \end{aligned} \tag{2.24}$$

in which Ψ, O and $\boldsymbol{p}$ are expressed by their real and imaginary components, ψ_i is the basis function, < > indicates integration over the problem domain and the second-order absorption boundary conditions are employed here (Yuan *et al* 2006),

$$\nabla\psi_n \cdot \hat{n} = \eta\psi_n + \gamma\frac{\partial^2\psi_n}{\partial^2\theta} \tag{2.25}$$

where $\eta = \frac{-ik - 3/2\rho + i3/8k\rho^2}{1 - i/k\rho}$, $\gamma = \frac{-i/2k\rho^2}{1 - i/k\rho}$ and θ is the angular coordinate at a radial position ρ. To obtain a matrix equation capable of inverse solution, a combined Marquardt and Tikhonov regularization scheme is used for the inverse calculation,

$$(\Im^T\Im + \lambda\boldsymbol{I})\Delta\chi = \Im^T(\boldsymbol{p}^o - \boldsymbol{p}^c) \tag{2.26}$$

where $\boldsymbol{p}^o = (p_1^o, p_2^o, \ldots, p_M^o)^T$, $\boldsymbol{p}^c = (p_1^c, p_2^c, \ldots, p_M^c)^T$, and p_i^o and p_i^c are observed and computed complex acoustic field data for $i = 1, 2\ldots, M$ boundary measurement locations, $\Delta\chi$ is the update vector for the dielectric and acoustic properties, $\mathfrak{J}$ is the Jacobian matrix formed at the boundary measurement sites, λ is a scalar and $\mathbf{I}$ is the identity matrix. Thus, here the image formation task is to update dielectric and acoustic property distributions via iterative solution of equations (2.23) and (2.26) so that a weighted sum of the squared difference between computed and measured acoustic pressure can be minimized.

2.3 Simultaneous recovery of conductivity and elasticity

Adapted from Zheng and Jiang (2019).

Elastic modulus of tissue is an important parameter in disease diagnosis (Ophir *et al* 1991, Majumdar *et al* 1999), which can characterize tissue as soft or hard. At present, elastography has been implemented based on the contrast mechanism of ultrasound imaging (US) (Zaleska-Dorobisz *et al* 2014), optical coherence tomography (OCT) (Kennedy *et al* 2014), magnetic resonance imaging (MRI) (Mariappan *et al* 2010), or photoacoustic imaging (PAI) (Glatz *et al* 2015). These elasticity imaging techniques have been applied for the detection of liver fibrosis (Sandrin *et al* 2003), breast cancer (Itoh *et al* 2006) and prostate cancer (Cochlin *et al* 2002).

Here we add a new method to the family of elastography based on the contrast mechanism of thermoacoustic tomography (TAT). In thermoacoustic elastography (TAE), we reconstruct the bulk elastic modulus distribution by solving the thermoacoustic (TA) wave equation without internal or external static stress or shear wave. Our TAE approach is tested and validated using both simulated and phantom experiments.

2.3.1 Image reconstruction algorithm

Key to the realization of TAE is an image reconstruction algorithm based on the finite element method (FEM) that simultaneously reconstructs tissue energy loss and elastic modulus from tomographically measured TA signals.

Using Newton's law of motion, equation of continuity, and thermal elastic equation, the following time-domain TA wave equation can be derived (Jiang 2014):

$$\nabla^2 p(r, t) - \frac{\rho}{K}\frac{\partial^2}{\partial t^2} p(r, t) = -\frac{\beta}{C_p}\frac{\partial}{\partial t} H(r, t) \tag{2.27}$$

where p is the press wave, ρ is the mass density, t is the time, r is the spatial variable, K is the bulk elastic modulus, C_p is the specific heat capacity at constant pressure, and β is the thermal coefficient of volume expansion. H is the microwave excitation source term, which can be written as $H = \Psi(r)I(t)$, where $I(t)$ is the temporal illumination function and $\Psi(r)$ is the absorbed energy density. To obtain equation (2.1), a homogeneous elastic reference medium is assumed with density, $\rho = \rho_0$, and the bulk elastic modulus is denoted as $K = \rho v^2$, where v is the acoustic velocity. If we let $O = \frac{\rho_0}{K}$, and expand p and O as the sum of coefficients multiplied by a set of the basis function ψ_j and ψ_k, i.e. $p = \sum \psi_j p_j$ and $\mathrm{O} = \sum \psi_k O_k$, then the finite-element discretization of equation (2.27) is expressed as

$$\sum_{j=1}^{N} p_j\left[\int_s \nabla\psi_i\cdot\nabla\psi_j ds\right] + \sum_{j=1}^{N} \ddot{p}_j\left[\int_s \psi_i\psi_j\psi_k O_k ds\right] - \oint_l \psi_i \nabla p \cdot \hat{n} dl = \int_s \frac{\beta\Psi}{C_p}\frac{\partial I}{\partial t}\psi_i ds \tag{2.28}$$

where $\hat{n}$ is the unit normal vector.

The Bayliss–Turkel radiation boundary conditions are employed here (section 2.1),

$$\nabla p \cdot \hat{n} = -\frac{1}{v_0}\frac{\partial p}{\partial t} - \frac{p}{2r} \tag{2.29}$$

In both the forward and the inverse calculations, the unknown coefficients Ψ need to be expanded in a similar fashion to p, as a sum of unknown parameters multiplied by a known spatially varying basis function. Thus, equation (2.28) can be expressed in the following matrix form in consideration of equation (2.29),

$$[K]\{p\} + [M]\{\dot{p}\} + [C]\{\ddot{p}\} = [B] \tag{2.30}$$

where $\{p\}_t$, $\{\dot{p}\}_t$, $\{\ddot{p}\}_t$ are the values of the pressure and its derivatives at time t and the elements of the matrix are written as

$$K_{ij} = \int_s \nabla\psi_i\cdot\nabla\psi_j ds + \frac{1}{2r}\oint_l \psi_i\psi_j dl \tag{2.31a}$$

$$C_{ij} = \frac{1}{v_0}\oint_l \psi_i\psi_j dl \tag{2.31b}$$

$$M_{ij} = \int_s \psi_i\psi_j \sum_k \psi_k O_k ds \tag{2.31c}$$

$$B_i = \frac{\beta}{C_p}\int_s \psi_i\left(\sum_k \psi_k \Psi_k\right) ds \frac{\partial I}{\partial t} \tag{2.31d}$$

$$\{p\} = \{p_1, p_2, \cdots p_N\}^T \tag{2.31e}$$

$$\{\dot{p}\} = \{\dot{p}_1, \dot{p}_2, \cdots \dot{p}_N\}^T \tag{2.31f}$$

$$\{\ddot{p}\} = \{\ddot{p}_1, \ddot{p}_2, \cdots \ddot{p}_N\}^T \tag{2.31g}$$

Here, the Newmark's time stepping scheme is used for the discretization of the time dimension. To form an image from a presumably uniform initial guess of the microwave and mechanical property distributions, the iterative Newton's method is used to update Ψ and O from their starting values. In this method, we Taylor expand p about an assumed (Ψ, O) distribution, which is a perturbation away from some other distribution ($\tilde{\Psi}$, $\tilde{O}$), such that a discrete set of p values can be expressed as

$$p(\tilde{\Psi}, \tilde{O}) = p(\Psi, O) + \frac{\partial p}{\partial \Psi}(\tilde{\Psi}-\Psi) + \frac{\partial p}{\partial O}(\tilde{O}-O) + \cdots \tag{2.32}$$

If the assumed microwave/mechanical property distributions are close to the true profiles, the left-hand side of equation (2.32) can be considered as the true data (observed or measured), and the relationship can be truncated to yield

$$J\Delta\chi = p^o - p^c \tag{2.33}$$

where

$$J = \begin{bmatrix} \frac{\partial p_1}{\partial O_1} & \cdots & \frac{\partial p_1}{\partial O_K} & \frac{\partial p_1}{\partial \Psi_1} & \cdots & \frac{\partial p_1}{\partial \Psi_K} \\ \frac{\partial p_2}{\partial O_1} & \cdots & \frac{\partial p_2}{\partial O_K} & \frac{\partial p_2}{\partial \Psi_1} & \cdots & \frac{\partial p_2}{\partial \Psi_K} \\ \vdots & \ddots & \vdots & \vdots & \ddots & \vdots \\ \frac{\partial p_M}{\partial O_1} & \cdots & \frac{\partial p_M}{\partial O_K} & \frac{\partial p_M}{\partial \Psi_1} & \cdots & \frac{\partial p_M}{\partial \Psi_K} \end{bmatrix} \tag{2.34a}$$

$$\Delta\chi = (\Delta O_1, \Delta O_2, \cdots, \Delta O_K, \Delta\Psi_1, \Delta\Psi_2, \cdots, \Delta\Psi_K)^T \tag{2.34b}$$

$$p^o = \left(p_1^o, p_2^o, \ldots, p_M^o\right)^T \tag{2.34c}$$

$$p^c = \left(p_1^c, p_2^c, \ldots, p_M^c\right)^T \tag{2.34d}$$

and p_i^o and p_i^c are the measured and calculated acoustic field data based on the assumed (p, Ψ) distribution data for $i = 1, 2, \cdots, M$ boundary locations. O_k and Ψ_k $(k = 1, 2, \cdots, K)$ are the reconstruction parameters for the elastic and microwave property profiles, respectively. In order to realize an invertible system of equations for $\Delta\chi$, equation (2.33) is left multiplied by the transpose of J to produce

$$(J^T J + \lambda I)\Delta\chi = J^T(p^o - p^c) \tag{2.35}$$

where regularization schemes are invoked to stabilize the decomposition of $J^T J$. **I** is the identity matrix, and λ is the regularization scheme. The process now involves determining the calculated hybrid regularization-based Newton's method to update an initial microwave/elastic property distribution iteratively via the solution of equations (2.30) and (2.35) so that an object function composed of a weighted sum of the squared difference between computed and measured acoustic pressures can be minimized.

Considering the fact that ultrasound transducers and signal amplifiers have bandpass characteristics, we added the Butterworth bandpass filter module in the iterative process to improve the accuracy of reconstruction. We conducted several simulations and phantom experiments to demonstrate the feasibility of the proposed TAE.

2.3.2 Numerical simulations

In the simulations, different contrast levels of elastic modulus and energy loss between the targets and the background were used. A circular background region with the radius of 20 mm contained three circular targets (3 mm in radius each), positioned at 9, 2, and 6 o'clock, respectively. The bulk elastic modulus and energy loss of the targets are listed in table 2.2. The reconstructed method was implemented based on a dual mesh scheme (see section 3.1, chapter 3) with 1584 nodes and 2986 elements of coarse mesh and 6153 nodes and 11 944 elements of fine mesh. Thirty iterations were required for a complete image reconstruction. Each iteration costed ~6 min on a 3.6 GHz Core processor with 20 GB memory.

2.3.3 Phantom experiments

The TAT system we used to demonstrate the reconstruction method is detailed in section 1.3, chapter 1. The only difference is that a single-element unfocused transducer (V323, Olympus, central frequency: 2.25 MHz, nominal bandwidth: 1.35 MHz) is used here. In the phantom experiments, agar-based tissue-mimicking phantoms are used as the investigation samples. The elastic modulus is varied by changing the concentration of agar, while the microwave energy absorption is changed by adding 4% salt to the phantom. In the experiments, we make 2% (2.28 GPa elastic modulus) and 6% (2.43 GPa elastic modulus) agarose phantoms (3 mm in diameter each) with the transform oil background (1.90 GPa elastic modulus) for TAE. To improve the signal-to-noise ratio (SNR), an average of 100 times are adopted during signal acquisition. The same FE meshes as the simulations are used for the reconstruction using the experimental data.

2.3.4 Results

2.3.4.1 Numerical simulations

The anti-noise ability of the algorithm is also tested. For cases 1, 2 and 3, 'measured' data without noise and with 30 and 20 dB SNR are used as the reconstructed input, respectively. In each case, the measured data is generated using the forward computation with the exact elastic modulus and energy loss distribution at 180 receiving/detection positions equally distributed along the boundary of the circular background region.

Table 2.2. The parameters of background and targets. Reproduced with permission, from Zheng and Jiang (2019), © AME Publishing Company

	Radius (mm)	Location	Elastic modulus (GPa)	Energy loss (a.u.)
Background			1.90	0.001
Target 1	3	9 o'clock	2.25	1.5
Target 2	3	2 o'clock	2.43	1
Target 3	3	6 o'clock	2.34	2

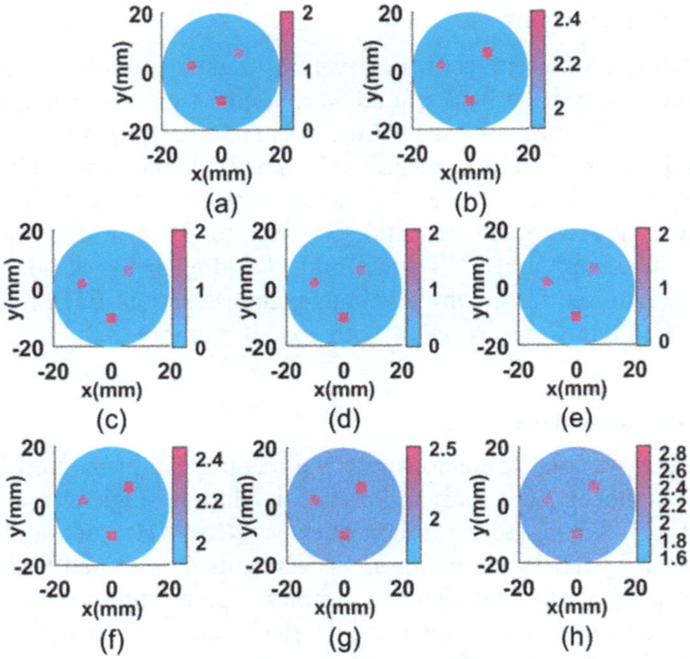

Figure 2.9. Reconstructed TAE images using simulations. Initial energy loss distribution (a) and elastic modulus distribution (b). (c)–(e) The reconstructed energy loss distribution for cases 1, 2 and 3, respectively. (f)–(h) The reconstructed elastic modulus distribution for cases 1, 2 and 3, respectively. Reprinted from Zheng and Jiang (2019), with permission, © AME Publishing Company.

Figure 2.9 shows the reconstructed images for simulation cases 1–3. We see that both the energy loss and elasticity can be well recovered for three targets having different contrast level relative to the background. When noise is added, we note that the energy loss can still be reconstructed with high accuracy, while the impact of noise on the quality of elasticity image is notable. To further quantify these observations, figure 2.10 is given to present the elastic modulus and energy loss profiles along the two transects crossing the centers of target 1 and target 2. We can see that recovered values of the targets match well with the exact values. The mean reconstruction errors of energy loss reconstruction and elastic modulus were found to be 0.15%/0.11%, 1.02%/1.77%, and 3.21%/5.49% for cases 1, 2 and 3, respectively.

2.3.4.2 Phantom experiments

Figure 2.11 presents the reconstructed TAE images and image profiles using the phantom experiments. From these images and image profiles, we see that our TAE algorithm has the ability to reconstruct energy density loss and elastic modulus simultaneously. The reconstructed shape and size of target agree well with the actual ones, and the error of the reconstructed elastic modulus compared to the exact value was estimated to be less than 3.3%.

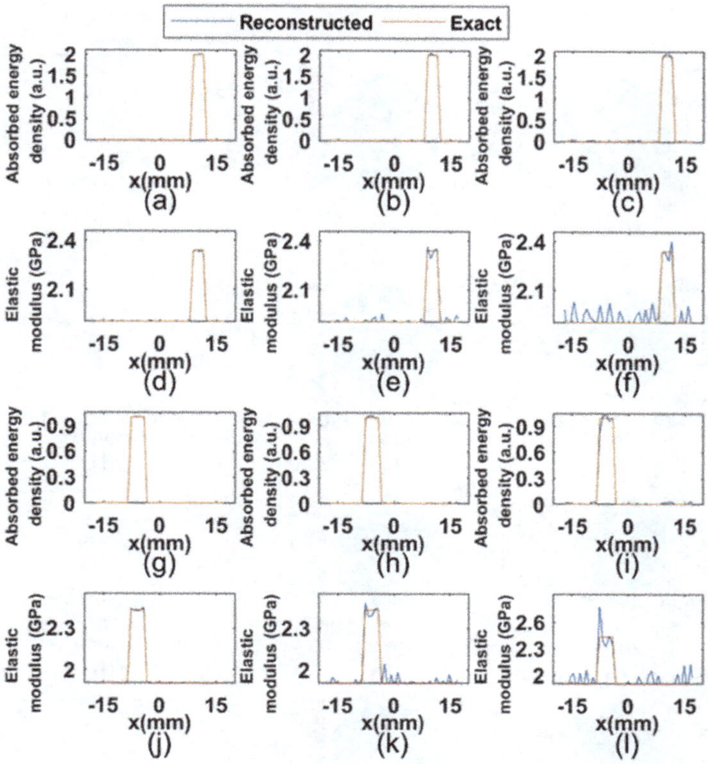

Figure 2.10. Comparison of the exact and reconstructed elastic modulus and energy loss along two transects crossing the centers of target 1 and target 2 for the images shown in figure 2.9. (a)–(c) Energy loss density along transects of the center of target 1 for cases 1, 2 and 3, respectively. (d)–(f) Elastic modulus along transects crossing the centers of target 1 for cases 1, 2 and 3, respectively. (g)–(i) Energy loss density along transects of the center of target 2 for cases 1, 2 and 3, respectively. (j)–(l) Elastic modulus along transects of the center of target 2 for cases 1, 2 and 3, respectively. Reprinted from Zheng and Jiang (2019), with permission, © AME Publishing Company.

2.3.5 Discussion and conclusion

Based on the results of simulation and phantom experiments presented above, it is clear that the image reconstruction algorithm described here is feasible. It has been demonstrated that the reconstructed images can provide both qualitative and quantitative information about the targets in terms of their location, sizes, shape, microwave and mechanical property values. These observations and the quantitative nature of the reconstructed images are further confirmed by the elastic modulus profiles provided.

From figures 2.9 and 2.10, we can see that both elastic modulus and energy loss distribution of the three targets with different contrast are accurately reconstructed. We note that the accuracy for the elastic modulus reconstruction is lower than that for the energy loss, especially when the SNR is reduced. The reconstructed elastic modulus given in figure 2.11 shows good agreement with the exact value. It is worth noting that the computational time for TAE image reconstruction is long at present.

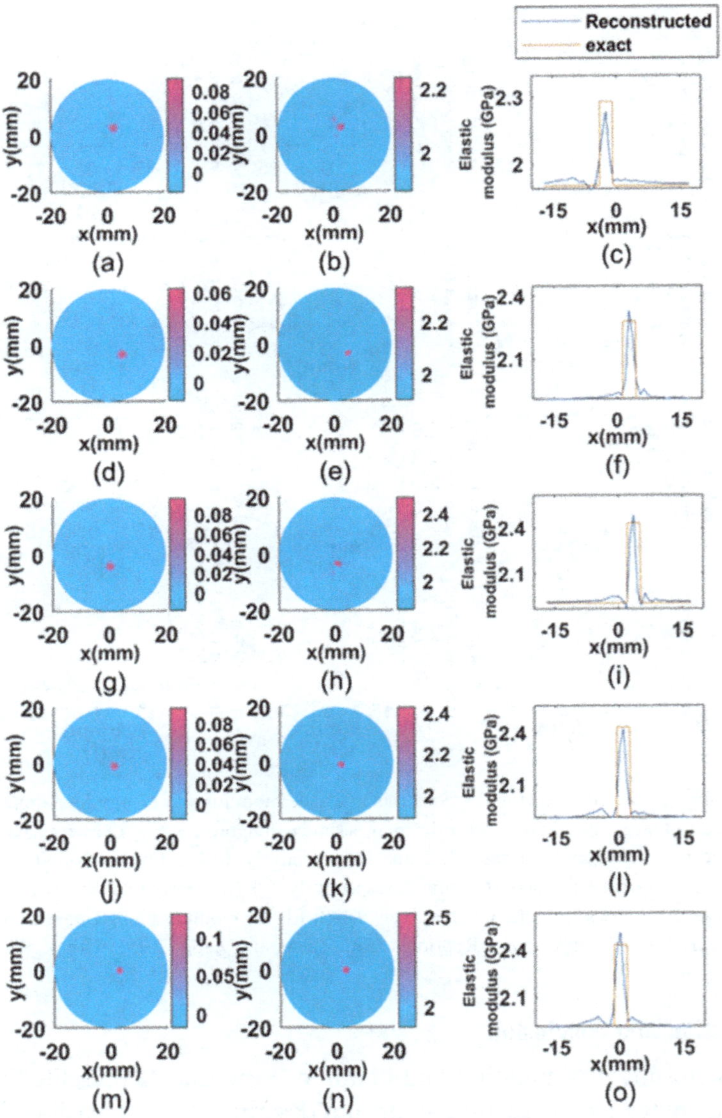

Figure 2.11. Reconstructed TAE images using experimental data. Energy loss density (left column), elastic modulus distribution (middle column), and the exact and reconstructed elastic modulus and energy loss profiles along transects crossing the center of each target (right column). Reprinted from Zheng and Jiang (2019), with permission, © AME Publishing Company.

This slow reconstruction process, however, can be speeded up using GPU-based parallel computing (see section 3.5, chapter 3).

In summary, we have demonstrated a TAE approach that allows the simultaneous recovery of elastic modulus and energy loss density using both simulated and experimental data.

References

Bayliss A and Turkel E 1980 Radiation boundary conditions for wave-like equations *Commun. Pure Appl. Math.* **33** 707–25

Ciocan R and Jiang H 2004 Model-based microwave image reconstruction: simulations and experiments *Med. Phys.* **31** 3231–41

Cochlin D L, Ganatra R H and Griffiths D F R 2002 Elastography in the detection of prostatic cancer *Clin Radiol.* **57** 1014–20

Glatz T, Scherzer O and Widlak T 2015 Texture generation for photoacoustic elastography *J. Math. Imaging Vis.* **52** 369–84

Greenleaf J F and Bahn R C 1981 Clinical imaging with transmissive ultrasound computerized tomography *IEEE Trans. Biomed. Eng.* **28** 177–85

Huang L, Yao L, Liu L, Rong J and Jiang H 2012 Quantitative thermoacoustic tomography: Recovery of conductivity maps of heterogeneous media *Appl. Phys. Lett.* **101** 244106

Itoh A, Ueno E, Tohno E, Kamma H, Takahashi H, Shiina T, Yamakawa M and Matsumura T 2006 Breast disease: clinical application of US elastography for diagnosis *Radiology* **239** 341–50

Jiang H 2014 *Photoacoustic Tomography* (Boca Raton, FL: CRC Press)

Jiang H, Yuan Z and Gu X 2006 Spatially varying optical and acoustic property reconstruction using finite element-based photoacoustic tomography *J. Opt. Soc. Am.* A **23** 878–88

Kennedy B F, Kennedy K M and Sampson D D 2014 A review of optical coherence elastography: fundamentals, techniques and prospects *IEEE J. Sel. Top. Quantum Electron.* **20** 272–88

Majumdar S, Lin J, Link T, Millard J, Augat P, Ouyang X, Newitt D, Gould R, Kothari M and Genant H 1999 Fractal analysis of radiographs: assessment of trabecular bone structure and prediction of elastic modulus and strength *Med. Phys.* **26** 1330–40

Mariappan Y K, Glaser K J and Ehman R L 2010 Magnetic resonance elastography: a review *Clin. Anat.* **23** 497–511

Mashal A, Booske J H and Hagness S C 2009 Toward contrast-enhanced microwave-induced thermoacoustic imaging of breast cancer: an experimental study of the effects of microbubbles on simple thermoacoustic targets *Phys. Med. Biol.* **54** 641–50

Mittra R and Ramahi O 1990 Absorbing boundary conditions for the direct solution of partial differential equations arising in electromagnetic scattering problems *Prog. Electromagn. Res.* **2** 133–73

Ophir J, Cespedes I, Ponnekanti H, Yazdi Y and Li X 1991 Elastography: a quantitiative method for imaging the elasticity of biological tissues *Ultrason. Imaging* **13** 111–34

Sandrin L *et al* 2003 Transient elastography: a new noninvasive method for assessment of hepatic fibrosis *Ultrasound Med. Biol.* **29** 1705–13

Smith I M and Griffiths D V 2004 *Programming the Finite Element Method* 4th edn (Hoboken, NJ: Wiley)

Yao L, Guo G and Jiang H 2010 Quantitative microwave induced thermoacoustic tomography *Med. Phys.* **37** 3752

Yuan Z, Zhang Q and Jiang H 2006 Simultaneous reconstruction of acoustic and optical properties of heterogeneous media by quantitative photoacoustic tomography *Opt. Express* **14** 6749–54

Zaleska-Dorobisz T, Kaczorowski K, Pawluś A, Puchalska A and Inglot M 2014 Ultrasound elastography—review of techniques and its clinical applications *Adv. Clin. Experiment. Med.* **23** 645–55

Zienkiewicz O C, Taylor R L and Zhu J Z 2005 *Finite Element Method:Its Basis and Fundamentals* 6th edn (Oxford: Butterworth)

Zheng Z and Jiang H 2019 Thermoacoustic elastography: recovery of bulk elastic modulus of heterogeneous media using tomographically measured thermoacoustic measurements *Quantitative Imaging Med. Surgery* **9** 4

Chapter 3

Image enhancement: software and hardware approaches

In this chapter, we describe a series of software approaches including dual meshing, adjoint sensitivity, total-variation-minimization (TVM), rigorous incident electric field, adaptive minimization strategy, and parallel computation to enhance TAT performance. These software approaches aim to improve image reconstruction in terms of forward and inverse solution accuracy, reduced noise effect, and computation speed. We also present several hardware approaches to improve the signal-to-noise ratio (SNR) and compactness of the TAT system.

3.1 Dual mesh scheme

Realizing the fact that acoustic fields at MHz frequencies change rapidly while tissue dielectric and acoustic/mechanical property distributions are usually relatively uniform, a dual meshing method is required for the iterative nonlinear finite element (FE)-based algorithms for fast yet accurate inverse computation. The dual meshing scheme exploits two separate meshes—one fine mesh for acoustic wave propagation and one coarse mesh for parameter recovery. This dual meshing scheme allows a significant reduction of the problem size during the reconstruction, thus increasing overall computational efficiency. In fact, the idea of dual meshing has been implemented in optical image reconstruction, where this method has proved to be able to significantly enhance the quality of image reconstruction (Jiang *et al* 1997, 1998, Gu *et al* 2003, Jiang and Yuan 2011). Here we present the implementation of this method in TAT reconstruction.

Implementation of the dual meshing scheme impacts two components of the reconstruction algorithm: (1) the forward solution at each iteration for the scattering pressure field where the acoustic and dielectric property profiles are defined on the coarse mesh while the forward solution calculation is based on the fine mesh, and (2) calculation of the Jacobian matrix which is used to update the acoustic and

doi:10.1088/978-0-7503-3163-0ch3

dielectric property profile estimates during the inverse solution procedure. Thus, for the forward solution, the inner product, $\langle(\cdot)\rangle$, e.g. in equations (2.23) and (2.24), is performed over the elements of the fine mesh, while O_R, O_I, Ψ_R and Ψ_I need to be expanded in the basis functions that are defined over the coarse mesh. For example, for an arbitrary node i of the fine mesh which is embedded in a coarse mesh element with nodes L_1, L_2 and L_3, the values of O_R and O_I at node i become:

$$\begin{aligned} O_R(x_i, y_i) &= \sum_{n=1}^{3} O_{R,L_n} \phi_{L_n}(x, y) \\ O_I(x_i, y_i) &= \sum_{n=1}^{3} O_{I,L_n} \phi_{L_n}(x, y) \end{aligned} \tag{3.1}$$

where ϕ_{L_n} is the Lagrangian basis function over the coarse mesh.

The second impact of the dual meshing method appears during the construction of Jacobian matrix, $\boldsymbol{J}$, which is used to update the object profile values. The elements of $\boldsymbol{J}$ are composed of the partial derivatives of the scattering field at the observation sites with respect to the values of O_R, O_I, Ψ_R and Ψ_I at each node within the coarse mesh. Considering the impact of the dual meshing, the elements of Jacobian matrix can be written as:

$$\begin{aligned} \partial A_{ij}/\partial O_{R,k} &= \left\langle -k_0^2 \phi_k \psi_i \psi_j \right\rangle \quad \partial A_{ij}/\partial O_{I,l} = \left\langle -ik_0^2 \phi_l \psi_i \psi_j \right\rangle \\ \partial A_{ij}/\partial \Psi_{R,k} &= \langle -ik_0 c_0 \beta \phi_k \psi_i / C_p \rangle \quad \partial A_{ij}/\partial \Psi_{I,l} = \langle k_0 c_0 \beta \phi_l \psi_i / C_p \rangle \end{aligned} \tag{3.2}$$

where k and ℓ are the nodes on the coarse mesh, ϕ_k and ϕ_ℓ are the basis functions centered on nodes k and ℓ in this mesh, and the inner products are still performed over the elements in the fine mesh. Since ϕ_k and ψ_i are defined on the coarse mesh and fine mesh, respectively, evaluating these inner products can be quite involved. A way to simplify these integrations is to generate the fine mesh from the coarse mesh by splitting the coarse elements into fine elements.

Examples

Two phantom experiments were conducted to test the dual meshing scheme. We employed single-target-containing phantom tests, aiming to validate the accuracy improvement in detecting the target when the dual mesh is used. Cases 1 and 2 had a single target having 3 and 5 mm in diameter, respectively, and the single target in both cases contained sodium chloride with Agar powder (2%) for solidifying the sodium chloride solution, providing $\varepsilon_r = 57$, $\sigma = 6.07$ S m^{-1} at 3.0 GHz for the target. Transformer oil ($\varepsilon_r = 2.3$, $\sigma = 0.01$ S m^{-1} at 3.0 GHz) was used as the background phantom. Figure 3.1 shows the reconstructed absorbed energy density images for the two cases with uniform mesh and dual mesh. We see that the target is clearly better recovered with the dual mesh ((a) and (c)) in terms of its shape and size over that with the uniform mesh ((b) and (d)) for both cases. We also note that the background region for both cases is more smoothly recovered using the dual mesh scheme compared to that using the uniform mesh.

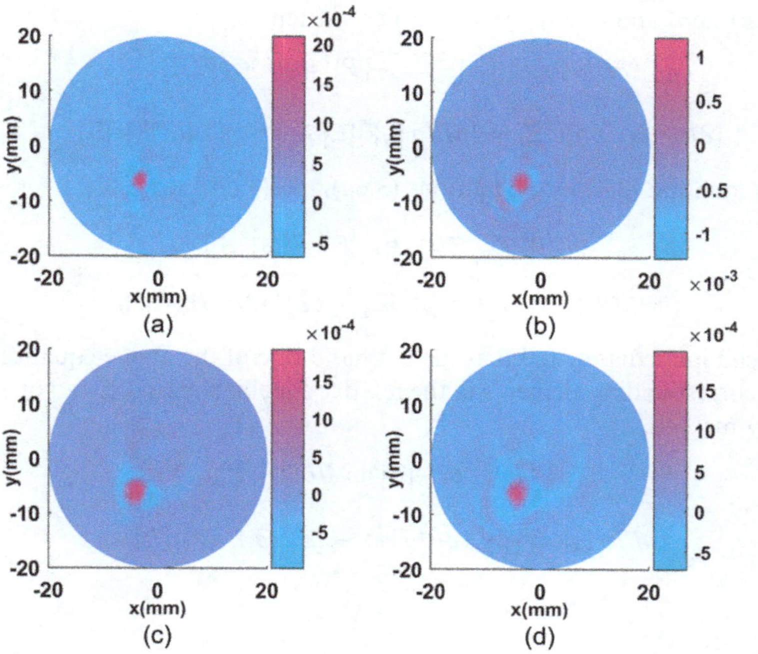

Figure 3.1. Reconstructed thermoacoustic images. (a) and (b) The image for case 1 with uniform and dual mesh. (c) and (d) The image for case 2 with uniform and dual mesh.

3.2 Adjoint sensitivity method

The coupled complex adjoint sensitivity method can be utilized to efficiently determine the Jacobian matrix (e.g. see equation (2.26)). Direct differentiation of both sides of equation (2.23) with respect to O_R and Ψ_R gives, respectively,

$$[A]\{\partial P/\partial O_R\} = -[\partial A/\partial O_R]\{P\} \tag{3.3a}$$

$$[A]\{\partial P/\partial \Psi_R\} = \{\partial B/\partial \Psi_R\} - [\partial A/\partial \Psi_R]\{P\} \tag{3.3b}$$

An equivalent set of equations can be obtained for differentiation with respect to O_I and Ψ_I by replacing O_R with O_I in (3.3*a*) and Ψ_R with Ψ_I in equation (3.3*b*). The Jacobian matrix can be calculated through the following steps:

First, we define a $\mathbf{N} \times \mathbf{M}$ matrix $\boldsymbol{\Xi}$, and let $\boldsymbol{\Xi}$ satisfy the following relationship:

$$[A]^T[\Xi] = [\Delta_d] \tag{3.4}$$

where the vector Δ_d has the unit value at the measurement sites/nodes and zero at other nodes. Then we left multiply (3.3*a*) and (3.3*b*) with the transpose of $[\Xi]$,

$$[\Xi]^T[A]\{\partial P/\partial O_R\} = -[\Xi]^T[\partial A/\partial O_R]\{P\} \tag{3.5a}$$

$$[\Xi]^T[A]\{\partial P/\partial \Psi_R\} = [\Xi]^T\{\partial B/\partial \Psi_R\} - [\Xi]^T[\partial A/\partial \Psi_R]\{P\} \tag{3.5b}$$

Equations (3.5*a*) and (3.5*b*) can be further written as,

$$\{\partial P/\partial O_R\}^T[A]^T[\Xi] = -\{P\}^T[\partial A/\partial O_R]^T[\Xi] \tag{3.6a}$$

$$\{\partial P/\partial \Psi_R\}^T[A]^T[\Xi] = \{\partial B/\partial \Psi_R\}^T[\Xi] - \{P\}^T[\partial A/\partial \Psi_R]^T[\Xi] \tag{3.6b}$$

Inserting equation (3.4) into equations (3.6*a*) and (3.6*b*), we get

$$\{\partial P/\partial O_R\}^T = -\{P\}^T[\partial A/\partial O_R]^T[\Xi] \tag{3.7a}$$

$$\{\partial P/\partial \Psi_R\}^T = \{\partial B/\partial \Psi_R\}^T[\Xi] - \{P\}^T[\partial A/\partial \Psi_R]^T[\Xi] \tag{3.7b}$$

Now we can immediately tell that the left hand side of the above equations actually gives the corresponding elements in the relative Jacobian matrix based on the adjoint sensitivity method,

$$\{\partial P/\partial O_R\} = -[\Xi]^T[\partial A/\partial O_R]\{P\} \tag{3.8a}$$

$$\{\partial P/\partial \Psi_R\} = [\Xi]^T\{\partial B/\partial \Psi_R\} - [\Xi]^T[\partial A/\partial \Psi_R]\{P\} \tag{3.8b}$$

3.3 TVM scheme

Measurement noises are always the major factor affecting the quantitative accuracy of the reconstructed images. In an effort to reduce the noise effect and to further enhance the quantitative accuracy of thermoacoustic image reconstruction, here we consider a TVM scheme within our FE-based reconstruction framework. Our existing reconstruction algorithms are based on the least-squares criteria (i.e. the regularized Newton method) (see chapters 1 and 2) that stand on the statistical argument that the least-squares estimation is the best estimator over an entire ensemble of all possible pictures. Total variation, on the other hand, measures the oscillations of a given function and does not unduly punish discontinuities (Dobson and Santosa 1994, van den Berg and Kleinmann 1995). Hence, one can hypothesize that a hybrid of these two minimization schemes should be able to provide higher-quality image reconstructions. In fact, the strategy of finding minimal total variation has proved to be successful in applications including electrical-impedance tomography (van den Berg and Kleinmann 1995), microwave imaging, image processing (Dobson and Santosa 1994), optimal design (Acar and Vogel 1994), and diffuse optical tomography (Paulsen and Jiang 1996).

A practical need exists for reconstruction of thermoacoustic images from few measurements, as this can greatly reduce the required scanning time and the number of ultrasound sensors placed near or on the boundary of an object to receive the microwave-induced acoustic signals. In addition, in many practical implementations of TAT the thermoacoustic signals are recorded over an aperture that does not enclose the object, which results in a limited-angle tomographic reconstruction problem. In such cases, the existing reconstruction algorithms, which are based on the least-squares criteria (i.e. the regularized Newton method) (see chapters 1 and 2), often generate distorted images with severe artifacts. It has been shown in photoacoustic tomography that the TVM-based algorithm offers excellent photoacoustic image reconstruction from few-detector and limited-angle data (Yao and Jiang 2011).

We describe the implementation of TVM within the FE-based reconstruction framework in time-domain. To form an image from a presumably uniform initial guess of the absorbed energy density distribution we need a method of updating Ψ from its starting value. This update is accomplished through the least-squares minimization of the following functional:

$$F(p, \Psi) = \sum_{j=1}^{M} \left(p_j^o - p_j^c\right)^2 \tag{3.9}$$

where p_j^o and p_j^c are observed and computed acoustic field data for $i = 1,2,\cdots M$ boundary locations. Using the regularized Newton method, we obtained the following equation for updating Ψ:

$$(\Im^T \Im + \lambda \mathbf{I})\Delta\chi = \Im^T(p^o - p^c) \tag{3.10}$$

where $p^o = (p_1^o, p_2^o, \cdots p_M^o)^T$, $p^c = (p_1^c, p_2^c, \cdots p_M^c)^T$, $\Delta\chi$ is the update vector for the absorbed microwave energy density, $\Im$ is the Jacobian matrix formed by $\partial p/\partial\Psi$ at the boundary measurement sites; λ is the regularization parameter determined by combined Marquardt and Tikhonov regularization schemes, and $\mathbf{I}$ is the identity matrix.

Two typical approaches exist for minimizing total variation: a constrained minimization through the solution of the nonlinear TA equation (Rudin *et al* 1992, Paulsen and Jiang 1996) and an unconstrained minimization by addition of the total variation as a penalty term to the least-squares functional (Dobson and Santosa 1994, 1996). From a computational standpoint, unconstrained minimizations are much easier to implement and require many fewer modifications to the existing algorithm (Dobson and Santosa 1996). Thus here the unconstrained TVM is used.

We now incorporate the total variation of Ψ as penalty term by defining a new functional (Yao and Jiang 2011):

$$\tilde{F}(p, \Psi) = F(p, \Psi) + L(\Psi) \tag{3.11}$$

Here

$$L(\Psi) = \int \sqrt{\omega_\Psi^2 \, |\nabla\Psi|^2 + \delta^2} dxdy \tag{3.12}$$

is the penalty term, ω_Ψ and δ are typically positive parameters that need to be determined numerically. The minimization of equation (3.11) proceeds in standard fashion by the differentiation of $\tilde{F}$ with respect to each nodal parameter that constitutes the Ψ distribution; simultaneously all these relations are set to zero. These steps lead to the following nonlinear system of equations

$$\frac{\partial \tilde{F}}{\partial \Psi_i} = -\sum_{j=1}^{M}\left(p_j^o - p_j^c\right)\frac{\partial p_j^c}{\partial \Psi_i} + V_i \qquad (i = 1, 2\cdots N) \tag{3.13}$$

where

$$V_i = \frac{\partial L}{\partial \Psi_i} = \int \frac{\omega_\Psi^2\left[\left(\sum_{k=1}^{N}\Psi_k\frac{\partial \psi_k}{\partial x}\right)\frac{\partial \psi_i}{\partial x} + \left(\sum_{k=1}^{N}\Psi_k\frac{\partial \psi_k}{\partial y}\right)\frac{\partial \psi_i}{\partial y}\right]}{\sqrt{\omega_\Psi^2\left[\left(\sum_{k=1}^{N}\Psi_k\frac{\partial \psi_k}{\partial x}\right)^2 + \left(\sum_{k=1}^{N}\Psi_k\frac{\partial \psi_k}{\partial y}\right)^2\right] + \delta^2}} dxdy$$

Similarly to equation (3.10), the following matrix equation for TVM constrained inversion can be obtained

$$(\Im^T\Im + R + \lambda I)\Delta\chi = \Im^T(p^o - p^c) - V \tag{3.14}$$

where

$$R = \begin{bmatrix} \frac{\partial V_1}{\partial \Psi_1} & \frac{\partial V_1}{\partial \Psi_2} & \cdots & \frac{\partial V_1}{\partial \Psi_N} \\ \frac{\partial V_2}{\partial \Psi_1} & \frac{\partial V_2}{\partial \Psi_2} & \cdots & \frac{\partial V_2}{\partial \Psi_N} \\ \vdots & \vdots & \ddots & \vdots \\ \frac{\partial V_N}{\partial \Psi_1} & \frac{\partial V_N}{\partial \Psi_2} & \cdots & \frac{\partial V_N}{\partial \Psi_N} \end{bmatrix}$$

and $V = \{V_1, V_2, \cdots V_N\}^{\mathrm{T}}$.

3.4 Rigorous incident electric field and adaptive minimization strategy

In chapter 2, we show that conductivity distribution could be recovered by an FE-based reconstruction algorithm coupled with the Helmholtz equation. However, an assumption of a uniform electromagnetic (EM) field distribution was made. In addition, calibration was required to estimate the microwave strength and boundary parameters. In this section, we describe an improved quantitative TAT (qTAT) method to remove the uniform EM field assumption and calibration process, the two limitations associated with our previous qTAT method, using an adaptive minimization strategy and the actual/rigorous inhomogeneous EM field distribution from the antenna waveguide used. To further optimize our new method, deionized water coupled with a dielectric matching layer was used to reduce the influence of microwave scattering.

In TAT, a waveguide is typically used as the antenna to deliver the microwave to the object via coupling medium (e.g. oil). In a waveguide, the electric field in TE_{10} mode can be written as:

$$E_x = E_z = 0 \tag{3.15a}$$

$$E_y = -\frac{i\omega\mu a}{\pi} A_{10} \sin\left(\frac{\pi x}{a}\right) e^{-i\beta z} \tag{3.15b}$$

where E_x, E_y, E_z are the electric field components in the x, y and z directions, respectively, a is width of waveguide, A_{10} is the amplitude constant in TE_{10} mode, and β is the propagation constant. Because E_y distribution is symmetric the propagation of microwave can be approximated to a two-dimensional plane with $y = 0$. Therefore, the incident electric field E_s can be calculated through the electric field distribution of the waveguide.

The electric field (E-field) distributions given by the two models are compared and shown in figure 3.2. Here, the E-field distributions obtained by CST® simulation software are regarded as the actual ones. We calculated the E-field distributions in x–y plane (see figure 3.2(b) and 3.2(c)), while the E-field distributions given by the uniformly distributed plane wave model (UDPW) and the two-dimensional (2D) waveguide transmission model (2DWT) are shown in figures 3.2(b) and (c), respectively. To quantitatively compare the two models, the E-field distribution profiles at $y = 0$ are shown in figure 3.2(d). From figure 3.2, we can see that the 2DWT model describes the E-field distribution more accurately than the UDPW model.

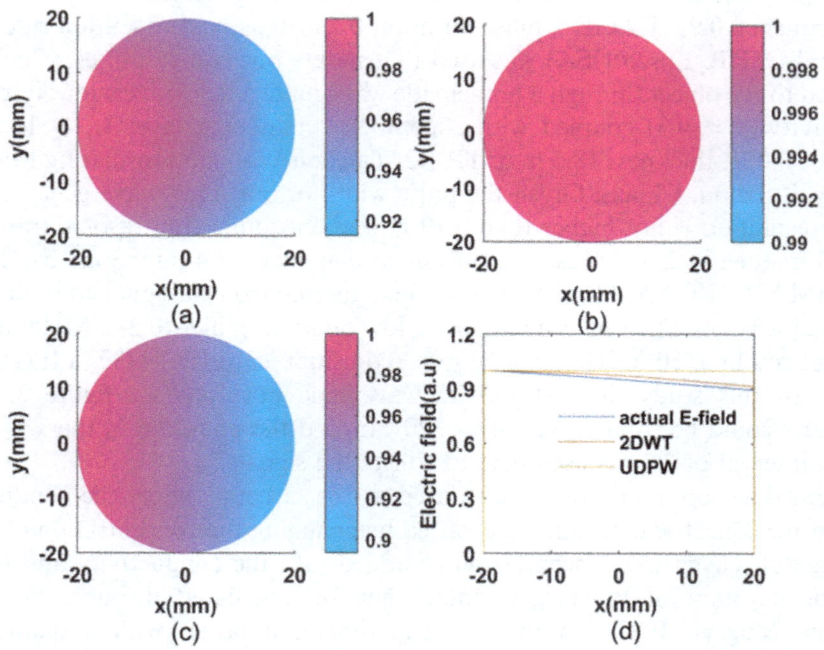

Figure 3.2. Comparison of the uniformly distributed plane wave model (UDPW) and the 2D waveguide transmission model (2DWT). E-field distributions given by the actual one (a), UDPW (b), 2DWT (c), and profiles (d) along a transect crossing the center in (a), (b) and (c), respectively. Republished with permission of Zheng *et al* (2020), permission conveyed through Copyright Clearance Center, Inc.

To eliminate the calibration procedure used in our previous qTAT algorithm, the following adaptive method is adopted here: (a) the energy loss distribution $s_r(\mathrm{r})$ is reconstructed using thermoacoustic signals; (b) estimate the possible range of conductivity σ_e and relative dielectric constant ε_e values of the object; (c) a series of energy loss distributions $s_{ij}(\mathbf{r})$ are calculated by substituting all the possible conductivity and relative dielectric constant values into equation (2.16) with E_s ; (d) calculate $\mathrm{err}_{ij} = \|s_{ij}(\mathrm{r}) - s_r(\mathrm{r})\|_2$; (e) steps (a)–(d) are repeated until a minimum is reached where conductivity distribution σ_c is obtained at the minimum. In this calculation, an average ε_e value of target is used. Furthermore, for experimental data, some pre-processing, including detrend, resample and threshold, was performed before the backprojection imaging reconstruction.

3.4.1 Simulations and experiments

We conducted several simulations and phantom experiments to test and validate the proposed a-qTAT approach. In the simulations, a single target with a diameter of 3 mm, a conductivity of 8.18 S m^{-1} and a relative dielectric constant of 62 was embedded in a background having 40 mm diameter, a conductivity of 0.001 S m^{-1} and a relative dielectric constant of 78. The simulation results obtained using both qTAT and a-qTAT are presented in figure 3.3. Furthermore, the err_{ij} during the calculation is shown in figure 3.3(f).

For the phantom experiments, a 1 GHz microwave generator (peak power 1–4 kW, frequency 0.95–1.2 GHz, pulse duration 0.25–50 µs, and repetition rate 20–25 000 Hz; PG5KB, Epsco USA) was used to generate microwave pulses, which were delivered to the object through a homemade waveguide filled with castor oil (relative permittivity $\varepsilon_r = 4.3$) coupled with a composite matching layer ($\varepsilon_r = 15.5$, loss tangent< 0.001, thickness 18.5 mm; TP-1/2, Taizhou Wangling Insulating Materials Factory, Taizhou, China). Given the pulse width of our microwave generator, the spatial resolution is not higher than 0.19 mm. A customized ultrasonic transducer (central frequency: 2.55 MHz, active-element diameter: 25.4 mm; 3 dB bandwidth: 100%; IMASONIC SAS, France)was used for thermoacoustic signal collection, and the signal was amplified by a home-made low noise amplifier (0.2–2 MHz, 60 dB), and digitized by a 50 MHz sampling rate acquisition card (PCI4732, VIDTS. Inc., China). In this study, limited by the waveguide position (see figure 3.4), the transducer could be rotated only over 320° around the phantom in the x–y plane, and, an interval of 2° was used here to collect the signals.

Here, saline-containing tubes were used as the target(s) where the conductivity and relative dielectric constant were varied by changing the concentration of salt in the target(s). Given the concentration of added salt, the conductivity and relative dielectric constant of the targets could then be calculated through the Debye equation (Stogryn 1971). In the first experiment, a target with a diameter of 3 mm, a conductivity of 8.18 S m^{-1} and a relative dielectric constant of 62 at 1 GHz was imaged. A single target was placed at different positions, and the resulting images at all the positions were then fused in a single image, shown in figure 3.5(a). It can be seen that the target is quantitatively recovered at these

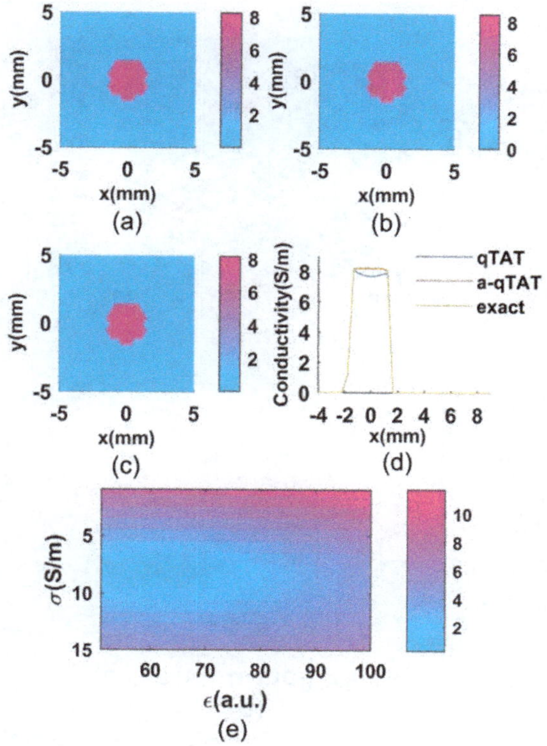

Figure 3.3. Simulations using a-qTAT and qTAT. The exact conductivity map (a), reconstructed conductivity distribution by qTAT (b) and a-qTAT (c). (d) Conductivity profiles along a transect crossing the background. (e) err_{ij} during calculation. Republished with permission of Zheng *et al* (2020), permission conveyed through Copyright Clearance Center, Inc.

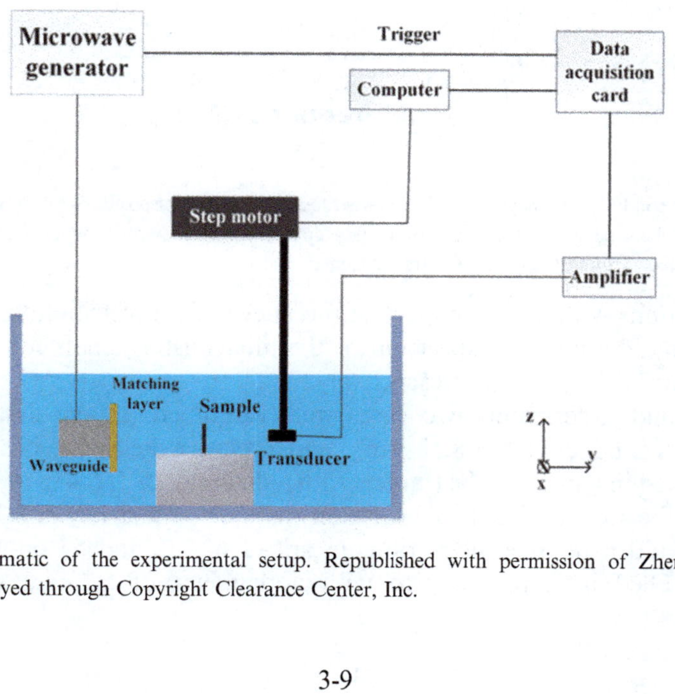

Figure 3.4. Schematic of the experimental setup. Republished with permission of Zheng *et al* (2020), permission conveyed through Copyright Clearance Center, Inc.

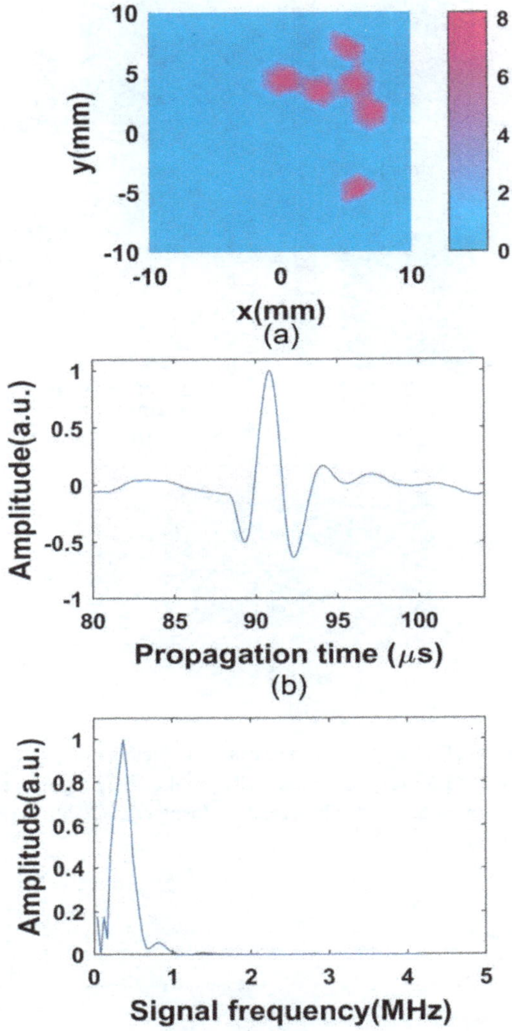

Figure 3.5. Fused conductivity image for a single target located at different positions (a), typical time domain and spectrum of thermoacoustic signal (b) and (c). Republished with permission of Zheng *et al* (2020), permission conveyed through Copyright Clearance Center, Inc.

different positions without the impact of the uneven field distribution. In addition, the typical time domain and spectrum of thermoacoustic signals for this case are shown in figures 3.5(b) and (c), respectively.

In the second experiment, two cases were examined. In the first case, NaCl solution with a conductivity of 8.18 S m^{-1} and a relative dielectric constant of 62 on 1 GHz was filled in a plastic tube (target) with a diameter of 5.2, 4.5 and 3.0 mm (see table 3.1). In the second case, NaCl solutions with a conductivity of 8.18, 12.57 and 10.45 S m^{-1} and a relative dielectric constant of 62, 52 and 57 on 1 GHz were, respectively, filled in a plastic pipe with a diameter of 5.2, 4.5 and 3.0 mm

Table 3.1. The parameters used for case 1. Republished with permission of Zheng *et al* (2020), permission conveyed through Copyright Clearance Center, Inc.

	Diameter (mm)	Position	ε	σ (S m^{-1})
Background			78.4	5.55×10^{-6}
Target 1	5.2	Top	62	8.18
Target 2	4.5	Middle	62	8.18
Target 3	3.0	Bottom	62	8.18

Table 3.2. The parameters for case 2. Republished with permission of Zheng *et al* (2020), permission conveyed through Copyright Clearance Center, Inc.

	Diameter (mm)	Position	ε	σ (S m^{-1})
Background			78.4	5.55×10^{-6}
Target 1	5.2	Top	62	8.18
Target 2	4.5	Middle	52	12.57
Target 3	3.0	Bottom	57	10.45

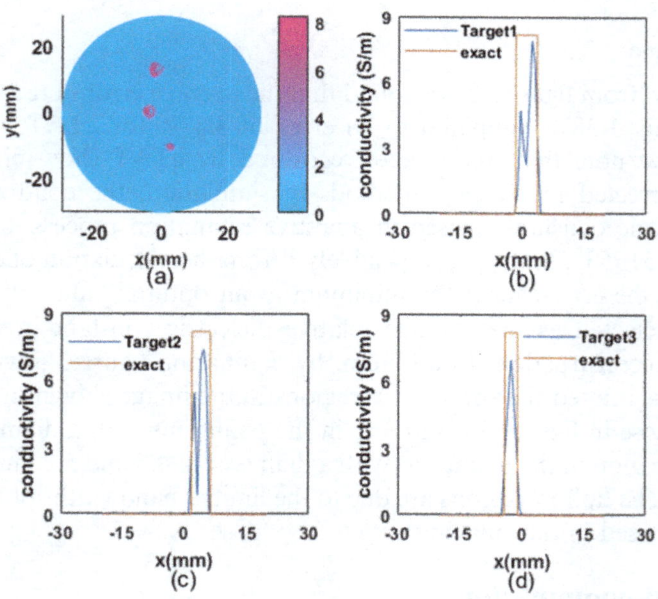

Figure 3.6. Reconstructed conductivity image (a) and profiles (b)–(d) for case 1. Republished with permission of Zheng *et al* (2020), permission conveyed through Copyright Clearance Center, Inc.

(see table 3.2). The conductivity images reconstructed by a-qTAT are shown in figures 3.6 and 3.7, respectively, for cases 1 and 2. We immediately note that the size and conductivity value of the target(s) are well reconstructed for both cases.

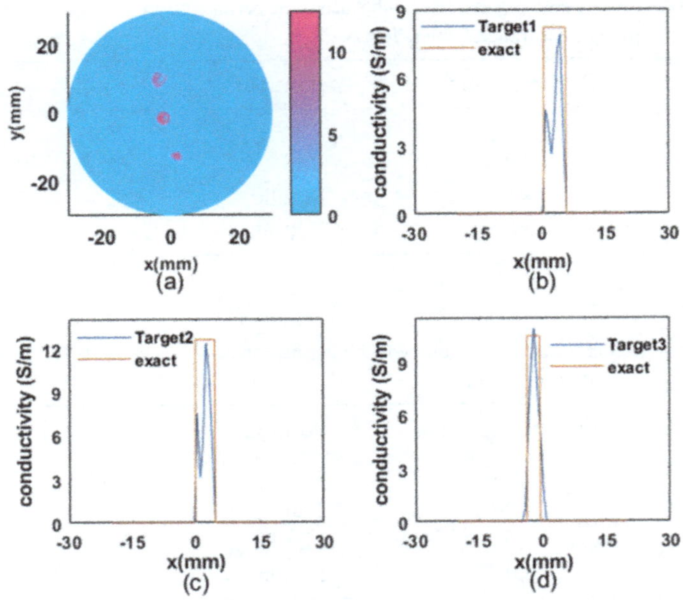

Figure 3.7. Reconstructed conductivity image (a) and profiles (b)–(d) for case 2. Republished with permission of Zheng *et al* (2020), permission conveyed through Copyright Clearance Center, Inc.

3.4.2 Discussion

Quantitatively, from figure 3.3, we found that the average error in reconstruction for a-qTAT is only 1.38% compared to an error of 4.87% for qTAT in simulations. Meanwhile, we note that, the images recovered by qTAT show pitting/artifacts, which are corrected in the new method. In simulation, the conductivity σ_e and relative dielectric constant ε_e used in adaptive estimation process are 1, 2, 3, …, 15 S m^{-1} and 51, 53, 55, …, 99, respectively. From the calculation of err_{ij} (shown in figure 3.3(e)), the err_{ij} reaches the minimum at an optimal value of ε_e. Therefore, $\varepsilon_e = 63$ was selected as the average relative dielectric constant in the target for conductivity reconstruction. In addition, by comparing figure 3.5 with figures 3.6 and 3.7, we also noted that no hollow regions in the image shown in figure 3.5 are larger than those in figures 3.6 and 3.7 (in the phantoms with a diameter of 3 mm, but a hollow region in the phantoms with a diameter of 4.5 and 5.2 mm versus 3 mm in diameter). The hollow regions are due to the limited bandwidths of the transducer and amplifier used in our imaging system.

3.5 Parallel computation

TAT image reconstruction in time domain, especially full 3D and large area reconstruction, requires significant computational times. Given the large problem size, in each discrete time step, the major areas of the algorithm are costly by dense matrix operations: (1) calculation of the derivatives of acoustic field with respect to electric/acoustic properties at the receiver sites, (2) buildup of the Jacobian matrix, which requires solving of linear equations, and (3) computation of a full matrix equation for the inverse solution. All the above processes involve massive calculation of a large dense matrix, which means that parallel computation can be adapted for TAT image reconstruction.

Graphic processing unit (GPU)-accelerated based on NVIDIA's Common Unified Device Architecture (CUDA) which provides a unified hardware and software solution for parallel computing is implemented here to achieve high computational speed of matrix operations. Before implementing the linear algebra library cuSPARSE, cuBLAS, and cuSolvers, which provide the linear algebra operations on matrix and vectors for sparse and dense linear systems from CUDA, the algorithm is vectorized or matrixed. The parallel computing process is simplified as three steps shown in figure 3.8: (1) The host (CPU) transmits the mesh parameters of FEM and experimental data to the device (GPU), (2) the device completes the reconstruction process including the forward and inverse solutions, and (3) The reconstruction results are transmitted from the device to the host.

Here we give a detailed description on the parallel computing based on GPU-accelerated. In time domain, there is a solution process of linear equations on the acoustic field in the forward solution process or derivatives of the acoustic field in the inverse solution process, resulting in a common coefficient matrix A. Compared with a dense matrix, a sparse matrix can not only reduce the memory consumption, but also accelerate the calculation. Fortunately, matrix A is a matrix with very high sparsity. In order to take advantage of this feature and to combine with the actual situation, we first perform LU decomposition for matrix A (A = LU), which maintains its sparsity. Afterwards, the lower triangular matrix L and the upper triangular matrix U of matrix A stored in the memory are used to solve the linear equations instead of inverting matrix A in the subsequent calculation process. In addition, to maximize the efficiency of GPU calculation, the calculation process is adjusted from double precision to single precision. Finally, with little impact on the calculation error, we greatly improved the speed of single reconstruction. Table 3.3 lists the computation times taken by CPU and GPU codes after three iterations with

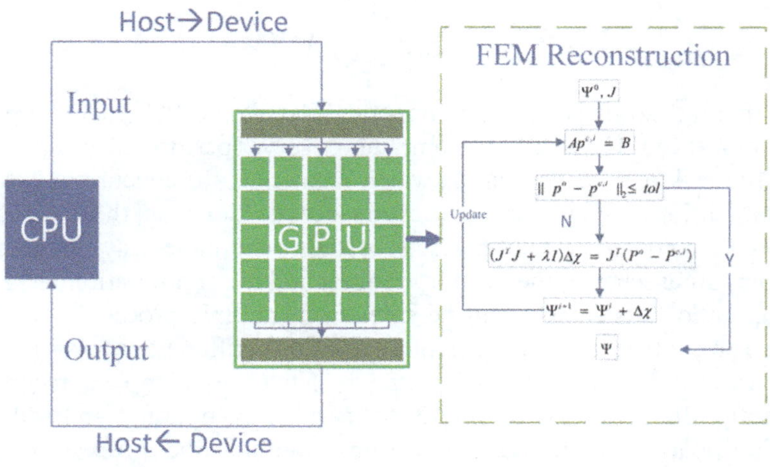

Figure 3.8. Schematic of parallel computing based on GPU-accelerated.

Table 3.3. Performance comparison between GPU- and CPU-based reconstructions. Republished with permission of Jiang *et al* (2019).

Dual mesh pair (nodes)	GPU (s)	CPU (s)	Acceleration ratio	Error
630–2457	2.13	370.11	173.8	<0.1%
930–3627	4.70	1504.00	320.0	<0.1%
1525–5977	13.50	7695.63	570.0	<0.1%
3542–13 973	135.80	80 006.50	589.1	<0.1%

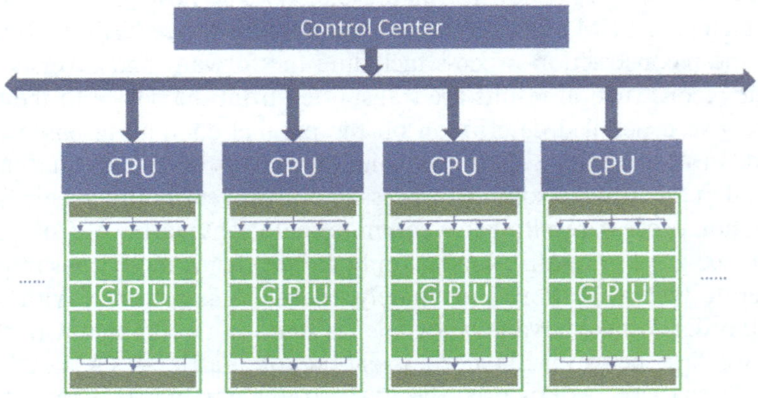

Figure 3.9. Schematic of multitasking in parallel computing.

respect to different mesh sizes, and corresponding acceleration ratio (i.e. the ratio between computation times of GPU and CPU). All the data was computed with a high-end GPU: NVIDIA TITAN x, and CPU: I7–4790k. A numerical comparison of the relative difference between the CPU- and GPU-based reconstructed results was conducted with the following equation:

$$E = \frac{1}{N}\sum_{i=1}^{N}\frac{|\Psi_{gpu,i} - \Psi_{cpu,i}|}{\Psi_{cpu,i}} \times 100\% \tag{3.16}$$

We see that the parallel computation method based on GPU greatly improves the reconstruction speed. However, the computer or server performance is redundant in general. Multitask parallel computing which is basically the concurrent execution of many computations using many processors can be done on the basis of GPU-accelerated to reconstruct multiple sets of data simultaneously. In a multitask parallel computing scheme, the memory request and the computation tasks of GPU for a computation assignment can be spread on multiple processors as shown in figure 3.9. The control center assigns multiple data to different processors, and each processor calls different GPU computing resources to complete reconstruction independently. In this way of multitask parallel computing and storage, the computation load and storage are assigned among the processors, and the computation assignment is maximally parallelized since each processor can run the assigned task independently without communicating with other processors. In addition, this method can be used to build data processing centers to reconstruct the data uploaded by multiple users at the same time.

3.6 Compact dipole antenna

Adapted from Huang *et al* (2018).

Although multi-channel data acquisition and transducer array-based thermoacoustic tomography (TAT) systems with a bulky antenna have been developed (Ye *et al* 2016, Ji *et al* 2015), at present it is difficult to translate them into clinical settings because the use of a bulky antenna allows very limited access to the tissue types/organ sites for thermoacoustic (TA) imaging. A TAT system with a portable antenna will permit TAT to be realized in reflection-mode, which could be used for imaging many tissue types/organ sites, or such a TAT system could also be conveniently utilized in an ambulance or bedside (Huang *et al* 2017, 2018). On the other hand, a portable TA excitation source is also important for a portable TAT system (see section 3.7). Herein, we describe a TAT system based on a handheld compact antenna coupled with a linear transducer array that would be better suited to clinical applications. We further investigate the effect of electric field attenuation, and determine the optimal attenuation compensation factor for the compact antenna.

3.6.1 Methods and materials

3.6.1.1 System description

Figure 3.10 depicts the schematic of a compact antenna based TAT system. To simplify the variables in a comparison of the handheld dipole antenna with

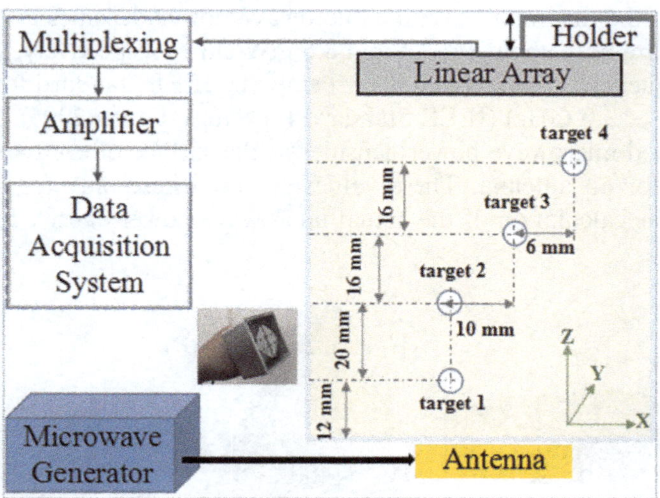

Figure 3.10. Schematic of the experimental system. Four 3 mm diameter tubes filled with 1% salt solution are located at different depths in the transformer oil-filled tank. The horizontal and vertical distances between the targets are given in the figure. The inset picture is the photograph of the handheld antenna. Reproduced from Huang *et al* (2018), with permission, © John Wiley & Sons.

the open-ended waveguide and pyramidal horn antenna, only transmission-mode (TM) TAT is used in this study (application of the handheld dipole antenna to reflection-mode TAT can easily be extended). Thus, in this system, pulsed microwaves with a center frequency of 3.0 GHz and a peak power of 70 kW radiate from a custom-designed magnetron generator are coupled to the antenna via a semi-rigid coaxial cable (1.5 m long with 1.2 dB insertion loss) to excite thermoacoustic (TA) waves (Huang *et al* 2012). The microwave pulse duration and repetition rates are 0.75 μs and 10 Hz, respectively. For TA signal collection, both the target to be imaged and a 128-element linear array transducer (5L128-I3, Olympus) are immersed into a transformer oil-filled tank to permit effective microwave/ultrasound signal coupling. The central frequency of the array is 5.0 MHz, with a bandwidth of 80%. The transducer-received TA signals are first transmitted into a 128–64 multiplexing system, then amplified via a homemade 64 channel amplifier, and finally acquired by two 32-channel data acquisition cards (NI5752, NI Inc. USA) at a sampling rate of 50 MHz (the signals are averaged 50 times to improve the SNR). Data processing and synchronization are simultaneously controlled by two onboard field programmable gate arrays (FPGA, 7972R, NI Inc. USA). Image reconstruction is performed using the delay-and-sum algorithm created by MATLAB (see section 1.2.1) (Hoelen and de Mul 2000).

3.6.1.2 Comparison between the compact antenna and conventional antennas

Three-dimensional models of the conventional open-ended waveguide, pyramidal horn antenna, and the handheld dipole antenna used in this study are given in figure 3.11. The dimensions of each antenna are: 34 × 72 × 200, 114 × 144 × 90 and 60 × 60 × 45 mm^3 (width × length × height) for the open-ended, pyramidal horn, and handheld dipole antennas, respectively. While the peak power of the microwave source is high, the maximum average microwave power densities at the surface of each antenna are only about 16, 3.1 and 8.6 mW cm^{-2}, respectively, when a 10 Hz repetition frequency is used, which is far below the IEEE standard for safety levels (20 mW cm^{-2} at 3.0 GHz) (IEEE Standard for Safety Levels 2005). Note that the above calculated microwave power densities at the surface of each antenna are the largest value for an antenna. These values are used here only for safety consideration, and the calculation of the actual microwave power density for an antenna

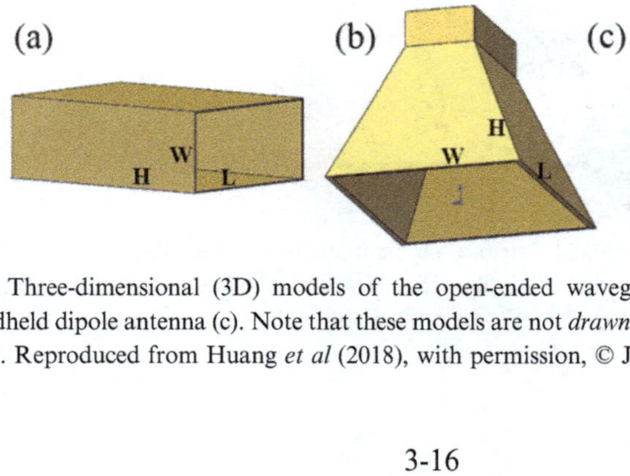

Figure 3.11. Three-dimensional (3D) models of the open-ended waveguide (a), pyramidal horn antenna (b), and handheld dipole antenna (c). Note that these models are not *drawn to scale*. *W*(*X*): width, *L*(*Y*): length, *H*(*Z*): height. Reproduced from Huang *et al* (2018), with permission, © John Wiley & Sons.

has to consider the impact of other factors such as the gain, directivity, efficiency, and effective aperture of the antenna.

Here, we note that the pyramidal horn antenna is physically the largest, while the open-ended waveguide is the longest as it is structured to achieve a high gain. In addition, as shown by the simulations given in figure 3.12, the rectangular apertures of the open-ended waveguide (a) and the pyramidal horn antenna (b) induce an ellipsoid radiation pattern. In contrast, the handheld dipole antenna yields a spherical radiation pattern due to its square/symmetric aperture, which is far better suited to imaging applications. Meanwhile, the field distributions of the dipole antenna in axial and vertical planes along with the far-field pattern are displayed in figures 3.12 (d)–(e).

3.6.2 Results and discussion

3.6.2.1 Results without electric field attenuation compensation

TAT imaging using both simulated and experimental data with the three antennas are conducted. The simulations are performed using the finite difference time domain (FDTD)-based electromagnetic (EM) software called CST (computer simulation technology), the experimental data are collected using the system shown in figure 3.10. In these simulations, four tubes, each with a relative permittivity of 70 and a conductivity of 1.85 S m^{-1} (mimicking a 1% salt solution) are input into the software accordingly (Huang *et al* 2012). The surrounding cube with a relative permittivity of 2.3 and a conductivity of 0.01 S m^{-1} is defined to mimic transformer oil (Engineering ToolBox (2010): Relative Permittivity-the Dielectric Constant; see https://www.engineeringtoolbox.com/relative-permittivity-d_1660.html). The simulated specific absorption rate (SAR) distributions of the four targets under these

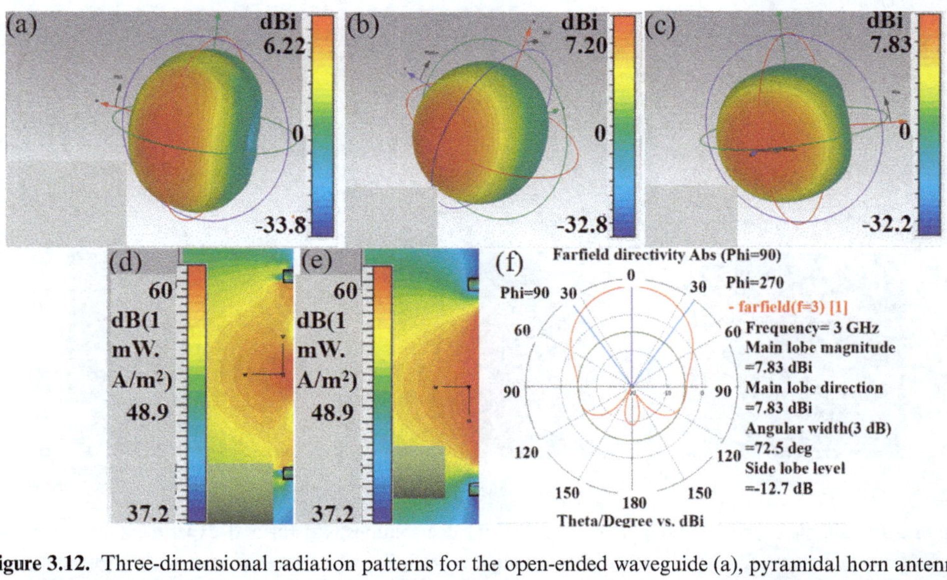

Figure 3.12. Three-dimensional radiation patterns for the open-ended waveguide (a), pyramidal horn antenna (b), and dipole antenna (c) generated with a commercial software called CST. Field distribution in axial (*YZ*) plane (d), vertical (*XZ*) plane (e) and the far-filed pattern of the dipole antenna. Reproduced from Huang *et al* (2018), with permission, © John Wiley & Sons.

different antenna illumination approaches are shown in figures 3.13(a)–(c), while the reconstructed TAT images using the experimental data are given in figures 3.13(d)–(f). We can see that the experimental results are in good agreement with the simulations.

3.6.2.2 Results with electric field attenuation compensation

We further calculate the Fresnel zone (***R***), which is the region of the field of an antenna between the reactive near-field region ($\boldsymbol{R}_1$) and the far-field region ($\boldsymbol{R}_2$). $\boldsymbol{R}_1$ and $\boldsymbol{R}_2$ are calculated using the following relationships (Balanis 2011)

$$\begin{cases} R_1 = 0.62\sqrt{d^3/\lambda} \\ R_2 = 2d^2/\lambda \end{cases} \tag{3.17}$$

where d is the largest dimension of the antenna, and $\lambda = 6.6$ cm is the wavelength in oil. Since the aperture size is given for the three antennas, we can obtain $\boldsymbol{R}_1 = 46$, 132 and 35 mm, and $\boldsymbol{R}_2 = 157$, 629 and 109 mm, for the open-ended waveguide, pyramidal horn antenna, and handheld dipole antenna, respectively.

We observe that for the open-ended waveguide and the handheld dipole antenna, targets (3,4) and (2,3,4) are located within the Fresnel zone, respectively, while no target is located within the Fresnel zone for the pyramidal horn antenna. As reported previously, the Fresnel zone field is defined as a $1/r$ field, and the electric field amplitude along the radiation direction can be approximately expressed as (Shackelford 1962)

$$E_\theta(r) \propto E_0/r \tag{3.18}$$

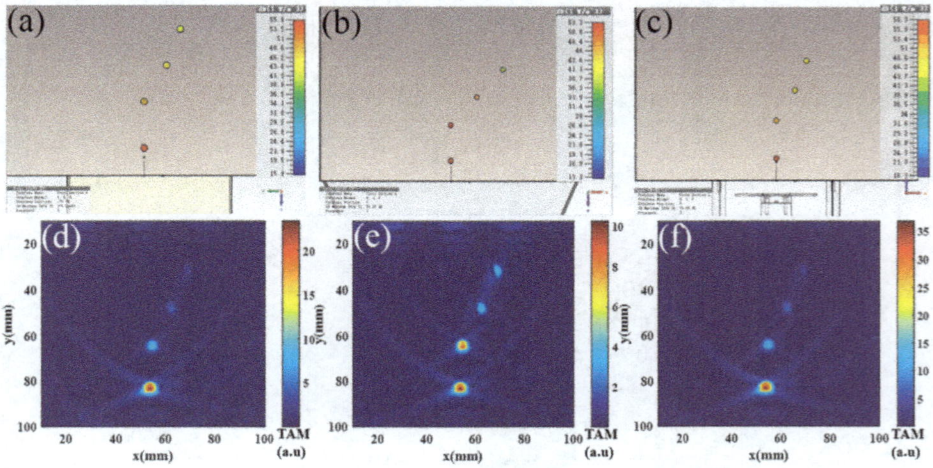

Figure 3.13. Simulated specific absorption rate (SAR) distributions, (a)–(c) and experimentally recovered thermoacoustic images, (d)–(f) of the 4 targets as indicated in figure 3.10, using the open-ended waveguide (a), (d), pyramidal horn antenna (b), (e), and handheld dipole antenna (c), (f) illuminations, respectively. TAM: thermoacoustic amplitude, a.u: arbitrary units. Reproduced from Huang *et al* (2018), with permission, © John Wiley & Sons.

where r is the distance between the antenna surface and the target (not the distance to the origin of the aperture surface), and E_0 is the electric field amplitude at the surface of the antenna.

For TA signal generation within the Fresnel zone, $E_\theta(r)$ is dominated. The initial TA pressure p_0 is the product of the deposited energy and the Grüneisen coefficient Γ of the tissue:

$$p_0 = \Gamma A(\vec{r}) = \Gamma\sigma(\vec{r}) \cdot E^2(\vec{r}) \tag{3.19}$$

where σ is the conductivity. We see that in this study the only difference is the electric field $E(\vec{r})$ for the four targets under different antenna illumination. Thus, p_0 can be expressed as:

$$p_0 = \Gamma A(\vec{r}) = \Gamma\sigma(\vec{r}) \cdot E^2(\vec{r}) = \Gamma\sigma(\vec{r}) \cdot E_0^2/r^2 \tag{3.20}$$

In table 3.4, we give the simulated SAR and the TA-recovered initial pressure amplitude of each target using these different antenna illumination conditions. We also calculate the squared ratio of two adjacent targets according to equation (3.20), with this value being used as an E-field attenuation factor for image reconstruction. We find that the experimental results are in good agreement with the simulated results for targets (3,4) and (2,3,4) under the Fresnel zone excitation using the open-ended waveguide and the dipole antenna, respectively. Although target 2 is out of the Fresnel zone for the open-ended waveguide according to equation (3.17), there is only 2 mm in distance between this target and the calculated boundary of the Fresnel zone. Thus, we can see that both the simulated SAR and the TA-recovered initial pressure amplitude of targets 2–4 decrease as a function of $1/r^2$ for the open-ended waveguide and the dipole antenna illuminations, which is consistent with that calculated using equation (3.20). As no target falls within the Fresnel zone of the pyramidal horn antenna, it is difficult to establish such a relationship within the reactive near-field region for this antenna. Nonetheless, if a target is located in the Fresnel zone of the pyramidal horn antenna, the electric field decreases as a function of $1/r$.

To reduce the significant distortion caused by the effect of microwave attenuation especially for deep tissue imaging, we seek to consider the microwave attenuation

Table 3.4. Comparison of the simulated SAR and experimentally TA-recovered initial pressure amplitude of each target under different antenna illuminations. Reproduced from Huang *et al* (2018), with permission, © John Wiley & Sons.

		Initial TA pressure (a.u)/Simulated SAR (a.u)			
No.	r (mm)	OW	DA	PHA	EF
1	$r_1 = 12$	23/358	37/651	10.5/140	
2	$r_2 = 32$	10/98	15/185	9/206	$(r_2/r_1)^2 = 7$
3	$r_3 = 48$	4.5/41	7/93	4/67	$(r_3/r_2)^2 = 2.3$
4	$r_4 = 64$	2.5/18	4/48	4.5/7	$(r_4/r_3)^2 = 1.8$

r: distance between the antenna and the target. a.u: arbitrary unit. OW: open-ended waveguide. DA: dipole antenna. PHA: pyramidal horn antenna. EF: electric field attenuation factor.

effect in the reconstruction algorithm. We correct the linear array-based delay-and-sum reconstruction algorithm (Huang *et al* 2012) using the attenuation factor $1/r^2$, and attempt to recover the TA images of targets 2–4 using both the open-ended waveguide and handheld dipole antenna illuminations. Briefly, the electric field attenuation can be corrected as follows: first, the TA images are recovered without compensation as shown in figures 3.14(a) and (c). Each column in figures 3.14(a)– (c) is multiplied by a position matrix with the same size, where each element of the position matrix is the square of the distance between the pixel and the surface of the antenna. Finally, we obtain the compensated TA images (figures 3.14(b) and (d)). The TA-recovered images of targets 2–4 before and after the E-field attenuation compensation are shown in figure 3.14. We see that the E-field attenuation effect is greatly reduced using the E-field attenuation factor. We also find that the handheld dipole antenna-induced initial TA pressure is about two times larger than that of the open-ended waveguide.

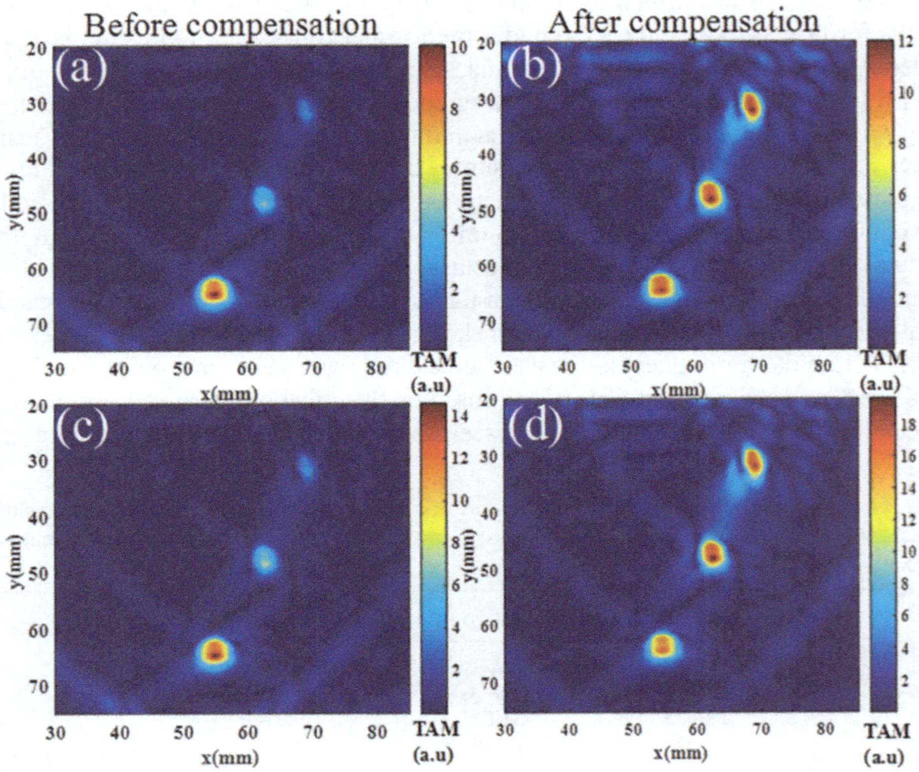

Figure 3.14. TA-recovered images of targets 2–4 using the open-ended waveguide (a), (b), and dipole antenna (c), (d) illuminations, before (a), (c) and after (b), (d) the E-field attenuation compensation. TAM: thermoacoustic amplitude, a.u: arbitrary units. Reproduced from Huang *et al* (2018), with permission, © John Wiley & Sons.

3.6.3 Conclusions

In this section, we describe a compact TAT system based on a handheld antenna. Compensation of the E-field attenuation for such a system is also achieved. One potential caveat of this proposal is that *in vivo* tissue has heterogeneous distributions of permittivity and conductivity compared to the simple targets used in the present study, making it harder to compensate the E-field attenuation accurately. Further *in vivo* evaluation of the compact handheld antenna in animals or humans is needed (see chapter 7).

3.7 Compact microwave source

The key component of a typical thermoacoustic tomography (TAT) system is a magnetron generator (MG) for thermoacoustic (TA) signal generation, and most TAT systems generally utilize a linear modulator-based high peak power MG for efficient TA signal excitation (Huang *et al* 2017, Zheng *et al* 2018, Nie *et al* 2010, Wang *et al* 2018). However, a linear modulator-based MG is bulky, and has dimensions of at least $850 \times 850 \times 1900$ mm^3 (width × length × height) with a weight of at least 150 kg (Huang *et al* 2017, Zheng *et al* 2018, Nie *et al* 2010, Wang *et al* 2018). In addition, it is expensive (up to \$70 000). Here we describe a lost-cost and compact MG-based microwave source that overcomes these limitations associated with the existing MGs. In this compact microwave source, the linear modulator is replaced by a solid-state modulator coupled with the associated electronics (Yin *et al* 2012). As shown in figure 3.15(a), the solid-state modulator-based MG is compact ($350 \times 210 \times 70$ mm^3 by volume) and low in weight (only 7.5 kg). The cost is also considerably reduced to \$40 000 or less. With this miniaturized MG, microwave pulses with a center frequency of 3.0 GHz, a peak power up to 60 kW and adjustable pulse duration from 70 to 600 ns can be generated to excite TA waves. The dimensions and weight of this MG are shown in figure 3.15(a) through the top and side views of the MG. Note that the MG's peak power, pulse duration and repetition rate are controlled by computer via two optical fibers. This compact MG and similar miniaturized MGs at other frequencies such as 1 and 2 GHz are now commercially available from Sichuan Huaweikang Medical Technologies, Inc. (Chengdu, China).

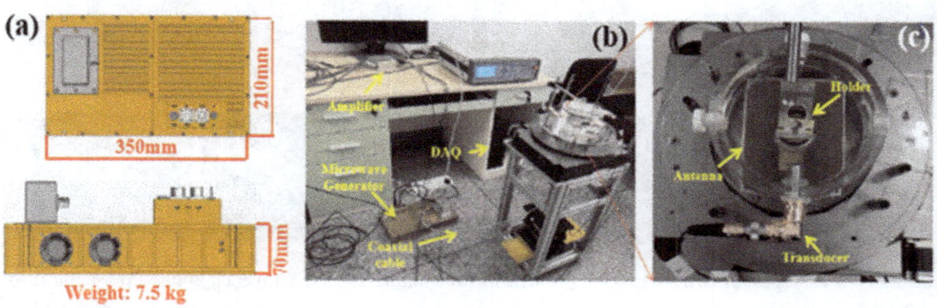

Figure 3.15. (a) Top and side views of the miniaturized MG. (b) Photograph of the TAT system. (c) Photograph of the antenna/transducer/oil tank interface. DAQ: Data acquisition.

3.7.1 Methods and materials

To demonstrate the performance of the miniaturized MG, a TAT system using a single scanning transducer is used. In the single scanning transducer-based TAT system (figures 3.15(b) and (c)), pulsed microwaves radiated from the miniaturized MG are coupled to a pyramidal horn antenna (114 × 144 mm^2) via a semi-rigid coaxial cable (1.5 m long with 1.2 dB insertion loss) to generate TA waves. A 5.0 MHz cylindrical focused transducer (V326, Olympus) rotates by a step motor detected the TA signals at 180 positions with a step of 2°. The transducer-received TA signals are first amplified by a pre-amplifier (Preamp 2-D, US Ultratek, Inc., USA), and then digitally acquired (PCI4732, Vidts Dynamic) after being averaged 50 times. In the experiments, both the sample and transducer are immersed in transformer oil for effective microwave/ultrasound signal coupling.

3.7.2 Results and discussion

3.7.2.1 TAT images of two crossed copper wires under different pulse duration
Several phantom and *in vivo* experiments are conducted to demonstrate and validate the imaging ability of the compact microwave source based TAT system. First, the TAT system is utilized to estimate the multiscale imaging potential of this system. Two crossed copper wires with a diameter of 150 μm each are thermoacoustically imaged under different pulse duration of microwave excitation, as shown in figure 3.16(h) (Razansky *et al* 2010). The reconstructed TA images of the two

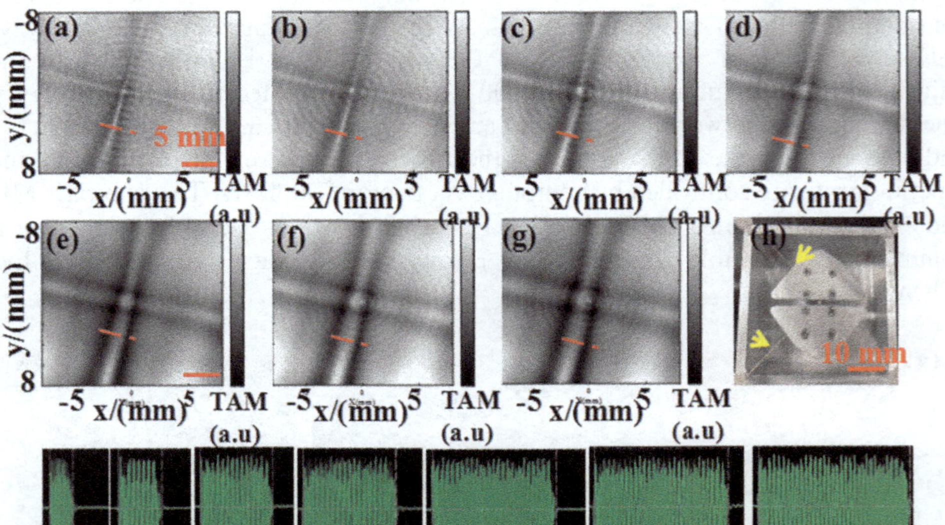

Figure 3.16. TA images for two crossed copper wires with a diameter of 150 μm each under a pulse duration of 70 ns (a), 170 ns (b), 270 ns (c), 370 ns (d), 470 ns (e), 550 ns (f), and 600 ns (g). (i)–(o) are the measured time-resolved pulse waveforms corresponding to (a)–(f), respectively. (h) is the photograph of the antenna and the copper wires (indicated by two yellow arrows).

copper wires under 70, 170, 270, 370, 470, 550 and 600 ns pulse durations are shown in figures 3.16(a)–(g). To monitor the stability and waveform of the MG, a power coupler (55 dB) integrated with the waveguide was used. Figures 3.16(i)–(o) present the time-resolved waveforms recorded by an oscillator (RTO1014, Rohde and Schwarz, German) that are utilized for producing the TA images shown in figures 3.16(a)–(g), respectively.

Table 3.5 gives the estimated full-width-at-half-maximum (FWHM) along the red dashed lines shown in figures 3.16(a)–(g). We can see that the diameter of the wire ranges from 0.3 to 1.4 mm as the pulse duration becomes longer, which is in good agreement with the theoretical prediction (Wang *et al* 2015, Lou *et al* 2011). Meanwhile, the frequency spectra of the TA signals obtained from figures 3.16(a)–(f) are given in figures 3.17(a)–(f). We note that a shorter pulse duration can generate TA signals with more high frequency components and provide higher resolution, which again agrees well with the theoretical prediction.

3.7.2.2 TAT images of in vivo *finger joint under different pulse duration*

To demonstrate the potential of the miniaturized MG-based s-TAT system for *in vivo* imaging, the proximal interphalangeal (PIP) of the right middle finger of a female volunteer is imaged. Figures 3.18(a)–(f) display the TA images obtained under 70, 170, 270, 370, 470 and 550 ns pulse durations. We compare the TA images with the 3.0 T MRI image for the same PIP joint of the volunteer (figure 3.18(g)),

Table 3.5. TA estimated FWHM of the copper wire along the red dashed lines shown in figure 3.16.

Pulse duration (ns)	70	170	270	370	470	550	600
TA-recovered diameter of copper wire (mm)	0.3	0.35	0.7	0.85	1.1	1.3	1.4

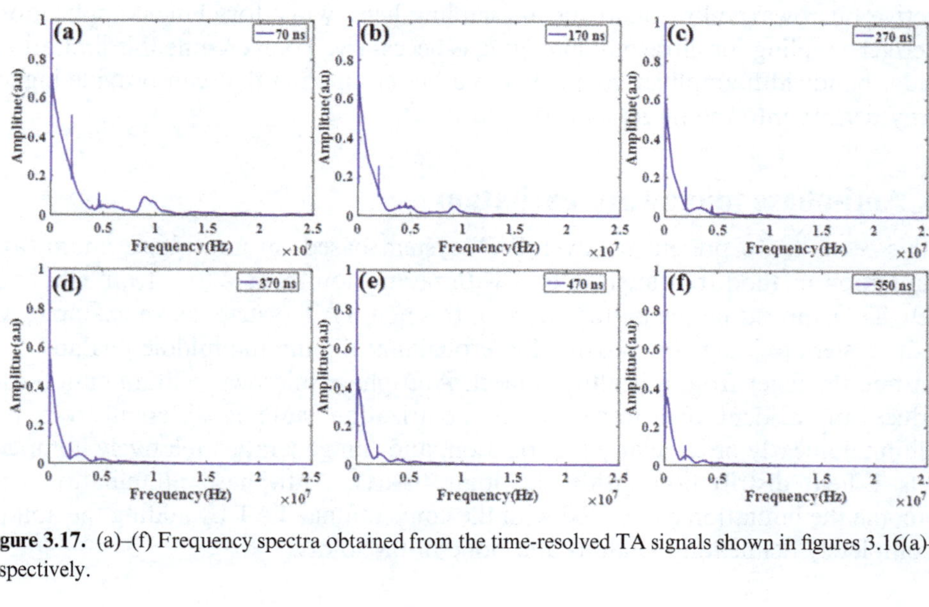

Figure 3.17. (a)–(f) Frequency spectra obtained from the time-resolved TA signals shown in figures 3.16(a)–(f), respectively.

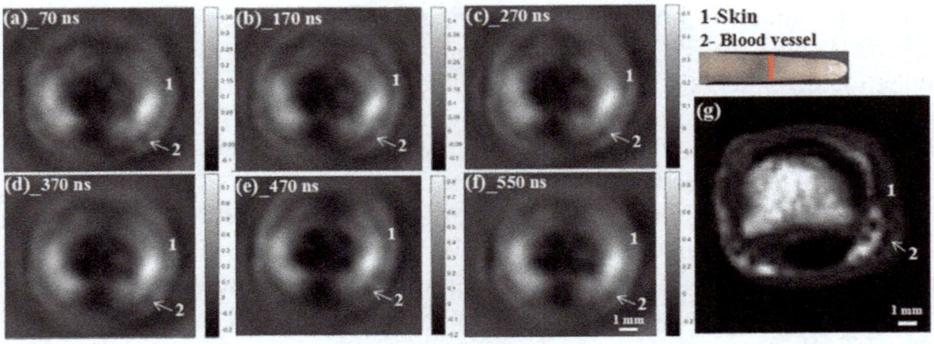

Figure 3.18. TA images of the PIP joint for a female volunteer under 70 ns (a), 170 ns (b), 270 ns (c), 370 ns (d), 470 ns (e), and 550 ns (f) pulse durations. (g) 3.0 T MRI image of the same PIP joint.

and notice that the TA image shown in figure 3.18(a) gives the best resolution where the skin (1), blood vessel (2), and some other joint tissues are identified.

3.7.3 Conclusions

In summary, a portable and inexpensive miniaturized MG, and thus a compact TAT system is described. It has been demonstrated that the miniaturized MG based TAT systems can be used for *in vivo* joint imaging with multiscale resolutions (0.3–1.4 mm). While the results presented are encouraging, there are still several improvements that need to be undertaken. For example, the spatial resolution of the TAT system is limited to ~1 mm[10] due to the limited bandwidth of the amplifier (−3 dB bandwidth: 0.5~2 MHz). Second, according to the experiment results presented, we note that the shorter the pulse duration and the lower per pulse energy, the weaker TA signals and worse SNR. In addition, transform oil is used for effective microwave/ultrasound signal coupling here, while for clinical application, water/gel coupling for ultrasound imaging is necessary. To overcome this limitation, a wider bandwidth amplifier coupled with a better antenna that can provide higher energy density into the target can be used.

3.8 Anti-phase microwave excitation

In this section, we present a novel TAT system based on anti-phase microwave illumination method (reprinted in part with permission from Wiley, from Chi *et al* 2019). To demonstrate the performance of this new TAT system, as an example, we use the system to image the proximal interphalangeal joint and middle phalanx of a right middle finger from a healthy subject. Anti-phase microwave illumination can produce an incident microwave whose polarization state is different from the traditional linearly or circularly polarization, and can generate a relatively homogeneous E-field distribution inside the joint tissues. Anti-phase illumination can overcome the limitation associated with the conventional TAT by adding the ability of completely delineating tendons and bone in the joints.

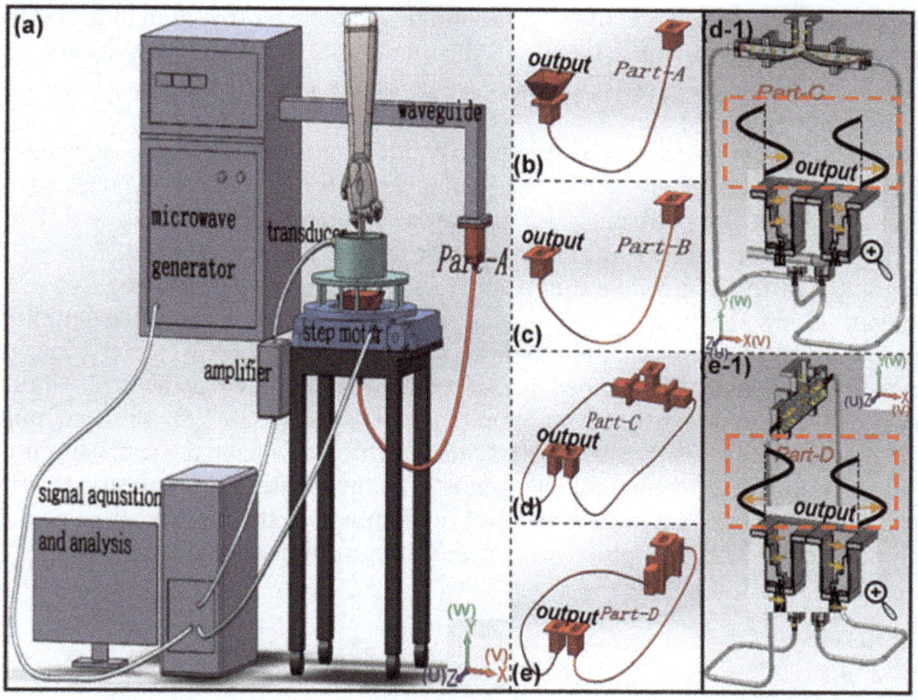

Figure 3.19. TAT imaging system, microwave illumination methods and simulations. Schematic of the system (a). Traditional microwave illumination (b) and (c): microwave output by a pyramidal horn antenna (b) and coaxial-to-waveguide adapter (c). Parallel in-phase microwave illumination (d): achieved by waveguide E-plane T-junction and coaxial-to-waveguide adapters. Parallel anti-phase microwave illumination (e): achieved by waveguide H-plane T-junction and coaxial-to-waveguide adapters. Simulations (d-1) and (e-1) correspond to (d) and (e), respectively. Reprinted from Chi *et al* (2019), with permission, © John Wiley & Sons.

3.8.1 Materials and methods

3.8.1.1 System description

The schematic of the experimental system is shown in figure 3.19(a). A pulsed microwave (frequency: 3.0 GHz, bandwidth: 50 MHz, peak power: 70 kW, and pulse duration: 750 ns) is delivered to the object/finger joint from the below vertically along the y-axis. The microwave power density at the object surface is measured to be less than the safety standard (100 W m^{-2} at 3 GHz). A 5 MHz cylindrically focused ultrasound transducer (V326, Olympus) is fixed to the organic glass cylinder (green color) filled with mineral oil. The transducer receives the acoustic signals at 180 positions (within 360°) via a step motor rotating the glass cylinder around the object. After being amplified by an amplifier, the signal is sampled and used for image reconstruction through the delay-and-sum method.

3.8.1.2 Microwave illumination methods

Four microwave illumination methods are given in figures 3.19(b)–(e). Through two coaxial-to-waveguide adapters and one coaxial connector (figure 3.19(b)), the high-peak-power pulsed microwave illuminates the finger by a pyramidal horn antenna with gain (figure 3.19(a)). If the pyramidal horn antenna is not used (figure 3.19(c)), the microwave can also shine to the object by a coaxial-to-waveguide adapter without gain.

Simulations using the two microwave illuminations methods depicted in figures 3.19(d) and (e) are presented in figures 3.19(d-1) and (e-1), respectively. These simulations are performed using Computer Simulation Technology software, and the simulation models are created according to the actual dimensions of the waveguides. In the microwave output port shown in figure 3.19(d), the two pulses propagate along the positive y-axis, and their E-fields have the same amplitude along the x-axis (i.e. in-phase illumination) shown in figure 3.19(d-1). Here, in-phase microwave illumination is defined because the two pulses reach the crest simultaneously. In the microwave output port shown in figure 3.19(e), the two pulses propagate along the positive y-axis, and their electric fields have the same amplitude but along opposite directions of the x-axis (i.e. anti-phase illumination) shown in figure 3.19(e-1). Here, anti-phase microwave illuminate is defined because one pulse reaches the crest while the other reaches the trough simultaneously.

3.8.2 Results

3.8.2.1 Electric field simulations

We first simulate the E-field polarization states of the incident microwaves radiated by the four microwave illumination methods. We then simulate the E-field distributions inside a layered cylinder finger model given the four microwave illumination methods.

The E-field polarization states of the incident microwaves radiated by the four microwave illumination methods are shown in figure 3.20. The simulation models are created according to the actual conditions as shown in figure 3.19, where the incident microwaves propagate along the positive w-axis. The incident microwaves radiated by the pyramidal horn antenna (figures 3.20(a) and (a-1)), by the coaxial-to-waveguide adapter (figures 3.20(b) and (b-1)) and by the in-phase illumination (figures 3.20(c) and (c-1)) are linearly polarized along the v-axis in the imaging area. However, the incident microwave radiated by the anti-phase illumination (figures 3.20(d) and (d-1)) has different state with the traditional polarization state. In the imaging area of $V > 0$ along the positive u-axis, most of the E-field rotates counterclockwise in the vuw plane. In the imaging area of $V < 0$ along the positive u-axis, the E-field rotates clockwise in the vuw plane. This difference can produce a new E-field distribution inside the finger to be imaged.

The finger model (80 mm in height) shown in figure 3.21(P) includes bones, ligaments/tendons, fat and skin. Dielectric properties of these healthy tissues at 3 GHz are assigned according to the literature (Gabriel *et al* 1996a, 1996b). We see that the E-field distributions generated by the pyramidal horn antenna (figure 3.21(a)), the coaxial-to-waveguide adapter (figure 3.21(b)) and the in-phase microwave illumination (figure 3.21(c)) are similar, and ‘cold spots’ appeared in

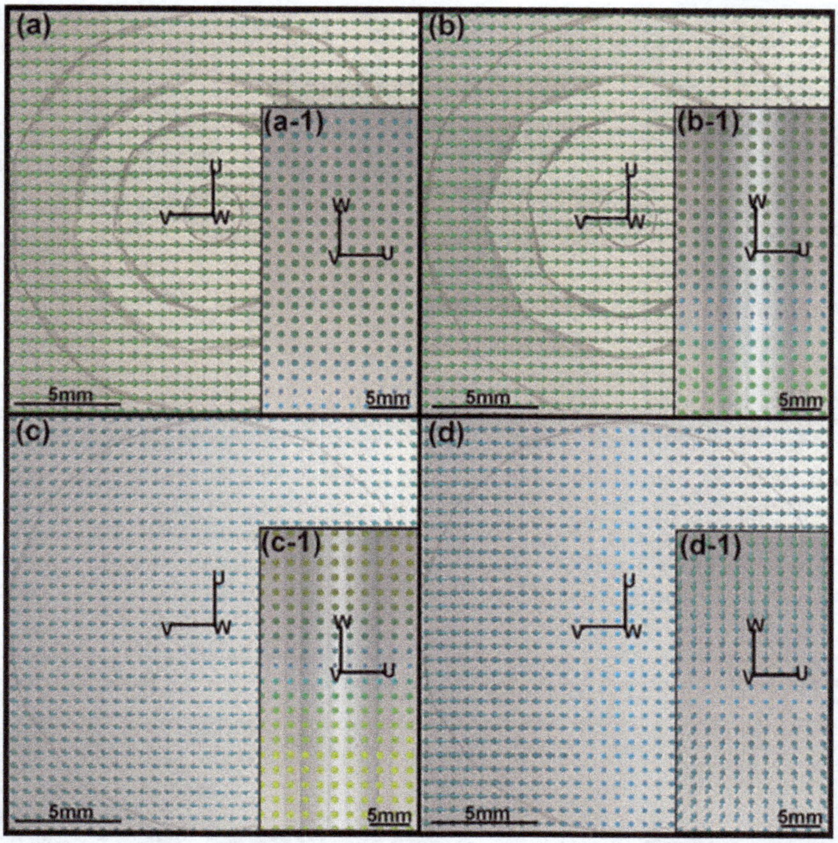

Figure 3.20. Simulated E-field polarization states of the incident microwaves radiated by the four microwave illumination methods shown in figures 3.19(b)–(e). E-field directions at some point in the cross sections along *w*-axis and along *v*-axis: microwave radiated by the pyramidal horn antenna (a) and (a-1); microwave radiated by the coaxial-to-waveguide adapter (b) and (b-1); parallel in-phase microwave illumination: (c) and (c-1); parallel anti-phase microwave illumination: (d) and (d-1). Reproduced from Chi *et al* (2019), with permission, © John Wiley & Sons.

these distributions. However, the E-field distributions generated by the anti-phase illumination (figure 3.21(d)) have no 'cold spots', and are relatively homogeneous.

3.8.2.2 TAT reconstructions

In this section, we present the TAT reconstructions of a proximal phalangeal joint for the four microwave illumination methods. Comparative analyses among TAT images are performed. To demonstrate the reproducibility, TAT images of a middle phalanx are presented and analyzed. In addition, a differential image and averaged images are provided to compare the information contained in the anti-phase TAT images and in-phase TAT images, and to simply correct field dependent distortions, respectively.

Figure 3.22 gives the TAT images of the proximal phalangeal joint of a right middle finger for a healthy subject using all four microwave illumination methods

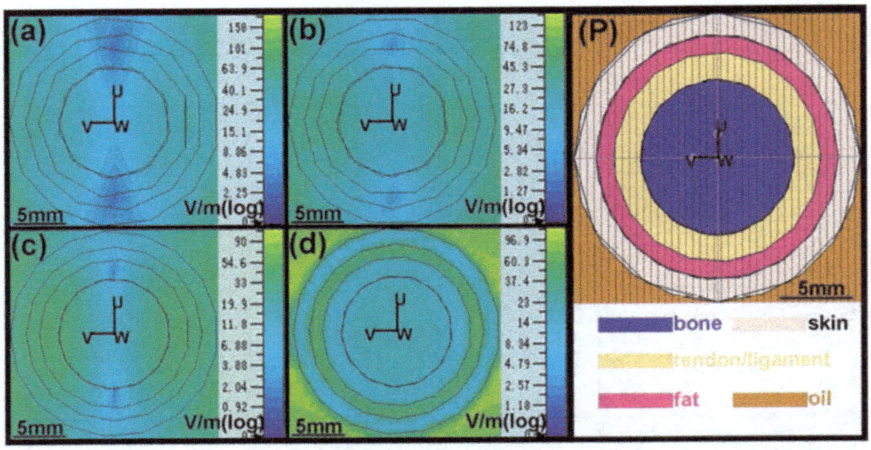

Figure 3.21. Simulated E-field distributions inside the layered cylinder finger model given by the four microwave illumination methods. The E-field distributions in the cross sections along the w-axis: microwave radiated by the pyramidal horn antenna (a); microwave radiated by the coaxial-to-waveguide adapter (b); the parallel in-phase microwave illumination (c); the parallel anti-phase microwave illumination (d). (P) is the layered cylinder finger mode. Reproduced from Chi *et al* (2019), with permission, © John Wiley & Sons.

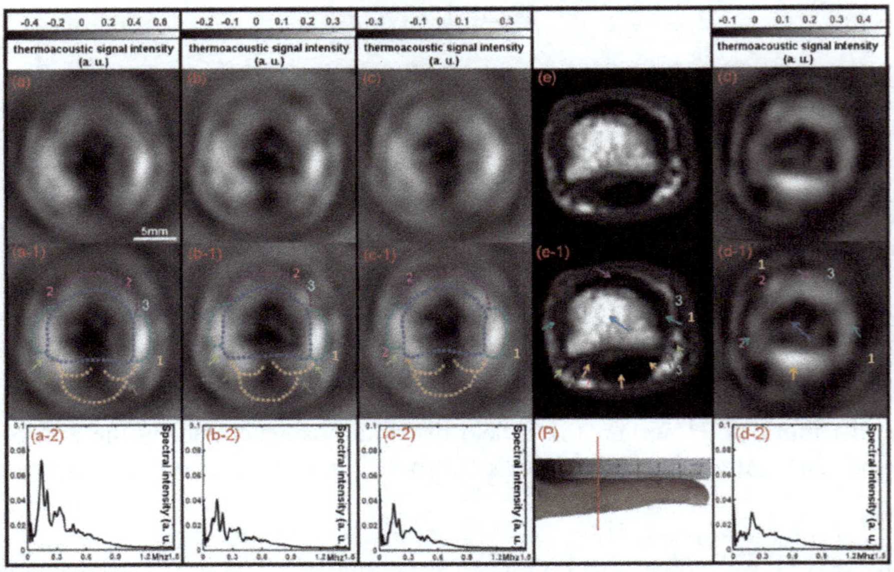

Figure 3.22. Cross-sectional TAT images of the proximal phalangeal joint of right middle finger for a healthy subject obtained by four different microwave illumination methods: by a pyramidal horn antenna output microwave (a) and (a-1), by a coaxial-to-waveguide adapter output microwave (b) and (b-1), by two coaxial-to-waveguide adapters with in-phase microwave (c) and (c-1), and by two coaxial-to-waveguide adapters with anti-phase microwave (d) and (d-1). MR image (e) and (e-1). The general outlines of the tissues for (a)–(e) are drawn in (a-1)–(e-1). The spectra for (a)–(d) are drawn in (a-2)–(d-2). (P) Photograph of the finger being imaged. Colored numbers and marks in some of the above images: 1-skin, 2-subcutaneous fat, 3-blood vessel, proper palmar digital artery, proper palmar digital nerve, flexor tendon, extensor tendon, collateral ligament, bone. Reproduced from Chi *et al* (2019), with permission, © John Wiley & Sons.

described in figure 3.19. For comparison, an MR image of the same joint is also given in figure 3.22(e). Based on the MR images, we draw different dashed lines along an alternate boundary between the light and dark regions in the TAT images. We see that the images by the pyramidal horn antenna (figure 3.22(a) and (a-1)), by the coaxial-to-waveguide adapter (figures 3.22(b) and (b-1)) and by the in-phase illumination (figures 3.22(c) and (c-1)) are almost identical and are able to identify various intra- and extra-articular tissues, including skin, subcutaneous fat, blood vessel, nerve, extensor tendon, collateral ligament, flexor tendon, and bone. However, the recovery of the bone and tendons is not complete, and some portions of these tissues are missing compared to the MR image. From figures 3.21(a)–(c), the extensor tendon and the flexor tendon are mixed with the 'cold spots', and cannot be completely reconstructed. Therefore, the inhomogeneous distribution of field can lead to significant deterioration of image contrast. Surprisingly, the images by the anti-phase illumination (figures 3.22(d) and (d-1)) give almost identical structure of the joint as compared to the MR image, and perfectly show the bone, flexor tendon, and extensor tendon, in addition other tissue types imaged by the other three methods. From figure 3.21(d), the extensor tendon and the flexor tendon can be

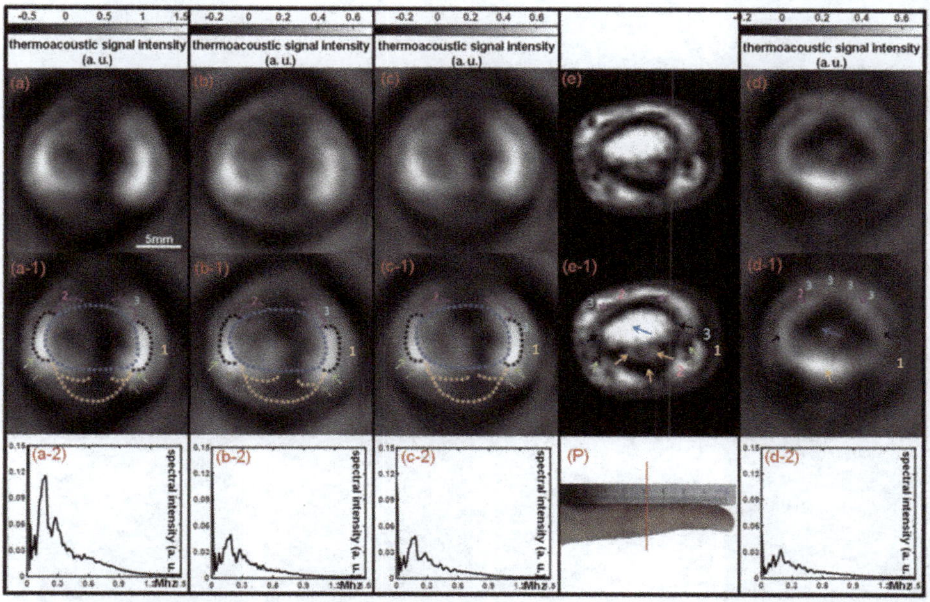

Figure 3.23. Cross-sectional TAT images of the middle phalanx of right middle finger for a healthy subject obtained by four different microwave illumination methods: by a pyramidal horn antenna (a) and (a-1), by a coaxial-to-waveguide adapter (b) and (b-1), by two coaxial-to-waveguide adapters with in-phase microwave (c) and (c-1), and by two coaxial-to-waveguide adapters with anti-phase microwave (d) and (d-1). MR image (e) and (e-1). The general outlines of the tissues for (a)–(e) are drawn in (a-1)–(e-1). The spectra for (a)–(d) are drawn in (a-2)–(d-2). (P) Photograph of the finger being imaged. Colored numbers and marks in some of the above images: 1-skin, 2-subcutaneous fat, 3-blood vessel, → proper palmar digital artery, → proper palmar digital nerve, → flexor tendon, → extensor tendon, → bone, → Retinaculum. Reproduced from Chi *et al* (2019), with permission, © John Wiley & Sons.

recovered completely and clearly, while the neighboring bony boundary is also recovered well.

Spectrum analysis is also presented. We first perform Fourier transform on the acoustic signal obtained by the transducer at each position (a total of 180 positions), and then add these signals to obtain a spectrum diagram as shown in figure 3.22(a-1). As mentioned in section 3.8.1.1, the acoustic signals at 180 positions are used to reconstruct the corresponding TAT image (figure 3.22(a)) through the delay-and-sum method. Therefore, the distribution of spectral intensity at different frequencies in spectrum diagram indicates the distribution of information contained in the TAT image at the corresponding frequency in frequency domain.

To further confirm the findings obtained from the images given in figure 3.22, cross-sectional TAT imaging of the middle phalanx of the hand is performed using the four microwave illumination methods (figure 3.23). Again, we see that the anti-phase method (figure 3.23(d) and 3.23(d-1)) gives the most information of the joint tissues and clearly reveal the bone, flexor tendon, and extensor tendon, in addition to other tissue types identified by the other three methods (figures 3.23(a)–(c) and 3.23(a-1)–(c-1)).

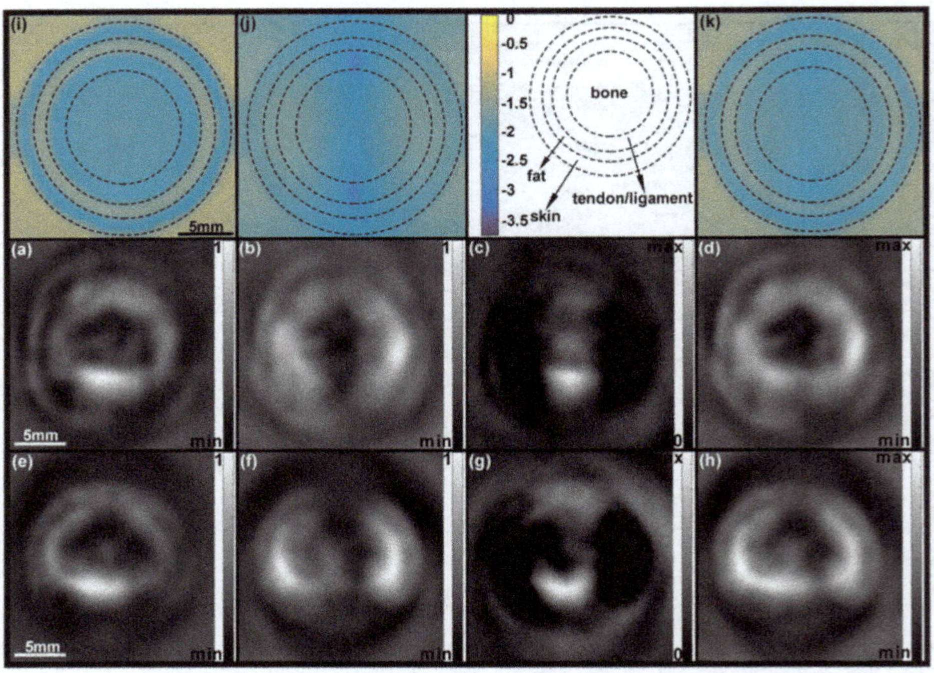

Figure 3.24. Differential image and averaged image reconstructions. Images in (a) and (b) are the normalized joint images given in figures 3.22(d) and (c), respectively. Image in (c) is the difference of (a) and (b). Image in (d) is the average of (a) + (b). Images in (e) and (f) are the normalized phalanx images presented in figures 3.23(d) and (c), respectively. Image in (g) is the difference of (e) and (f). Image in (h) is the average of (e) + (f). Normalized E-field distributions in the imaging cross sections: parallel anti-phase microwave illumination (i); parallel in-phase microwave illumination: (j); image in (k) is the average of (i) + (j). Reproduced from Chi *et al* (2019), with permission, © John Wiley & Sons.

To compare the information contained in the TAT images obtained by anti-phase illumination (figure 3.22(d)) and in-phase illumination (figure 3.22(c)), we first normalize these images to obtain the images given in figures 3.24(a) and (b) and then the differential image shown in figure 3.24(c) where the extensor and flexor tendon are highlighted. Figures 3.24(e)–(g) are obtained similarly. The E-field distributions for anti-phase illumination (figure 3.24(i)) and in-phase illumination (figure 3.24(j)) are also normalized. Compared with figure 3.24(i), the high E-field in the fat area is weakened in figure 3.24(k). Compared with figure 3.24(j), the effect of 'cold spot' in the tendon area is reduced in figure 3.24(k). The images shown in figures 3.24(d) and (h) are the averaged image of figures 3.24(a) and (b), and figures 3.24(e) and (f), respectively.

3.8.3 Conclusions

A TAT system based on anti-phase microwave illumination is described in this section. Using this system, it is shown that the anti-phase excitation can clearly and completely recover tendons and bone to overcome the limitations associated with the conventional TAT for joint imaging. However, limitations exist in this work. First, the adapters and connectors produce insertion loss when delivering microwaves. Such loss may lead to certain degradation of the SNR. To remedy the loss, two antennas with gain could be used to connect the adapters for outputting the anti-phase microwave. In addition, the mechanism on how the new E-field state of the incident microwave radiated by the anti-phase method affects the overall field distribution in tissue warrants further studies.

References

Acar R and Vogel C R 1994 Analysis of bounded variation penalty methods for ill-posed problems *Inverse Problems* **10** 1217–29

Balanis C A 2011 *Modern Antenna Handbook* (New York: Wiley)

Chi Z, Huang L, Ge S and Jiang H 2019 Technical note: antiphase-microwave illumination-based thermoacoustic tomography of *in vivo* human finger joints *Med. Phys.* **46** 2363–9

Dobson D C and Santosa F 1994 An image-enhancement technique for electrical impedance tomography *Inverse Problems* **10** 317–34

Dobson D C and Santosa F 1996 Recovery of blocky images from noisy and blurred data *SIAM J. Appl. Math.* **56** 1181–98

Engineering ToolBox 2010 Relative permittivity – the dielectric constant. See https://engineeringtoolbox.com/relative-permittivity-d_1660.html

Gabriel C, Gabriel S and Corthout E 1996a The dielectric properties of biological tissues: I. literature survey *Phys. Med. Biol.* **41** 2231–49

Gabriel S, Lau R W and Gabriel C 1996b The dielectric properties of biological tissues: II. measurements in the frequency range 10 Hz to 20 GHz *Phys. Med. Biol.* **41** 2251–69

Gu X, Xu Y and Jiang H 2003 Mesh-based enhancement schemes in diffuse optical tomography *Med. Phys.* **30** 861–9

Hoelen C G A and de Mul F F M 2000 Image reconstruction for photo-acoustic scanning of tissue structures *Appl. Opt.* **39** 5872–83

Huang L, Ge S, Zheng Z and Jiang H 2018 Technical note: design of a handheld dipole antenna for a compact thermoacoustic imaging system *Med. Phys.* **46** 851–6

Huang L, Li T and Jiang H 2017 Thermoacoustic imaging of hemorrhagic stroke: a feasibility study with a human skull *Med. Phys.* **44** 1494–9

Huang L, Yao L, Liu L, Rong J and Jiang H 2012 Quantitative thermoacoustic tomography: recovery of conductivity maps of heterogeneous media *Appl. Phys. Lett.* **101** 244106

IEEE Standard for Safety Levels with respect to human exposure to radio frequency electromagnetic fields 3 kHz to 300 GHz, IEEE Standard C95.1, 2005

Ji Z, Ding W, Ye F, Lou C and Xing D 2015 Shape-adapting thermoacoustic imaging system based on flexible multi-element transducer *Appl. Phys. Lett.* **107** 094104

Jiang H, Paulsen K D, Osterberg U L and Patterson M S 1997 Frequency-domain optical image reconstruction in heterogeneous media: an experimental study of single-target detectability *Appl. Opt.* **36** 52–63

Jiang H, Paulsen K D, Osterberg U L and Patterson M S 1998 Frequency-domain near-infrared photo diffusion imaging: initial evaluation in multi-target tissue-like phantoms *Med. Phys.* **25** 183–93

Jiang H and Yuan Z 2011 Photoacoustic tomography *Advances in Optical Imaging for Clinical Medicine* ed N Iftimia, W R Brugge and D X Hammer (New York: Wiley) ch 12

Jiang Y C, Zheng Z, Wang M and Yao L 2019 Total variation minimization enhanced quantitative microwave induced thermoacoustic tomography using a GPU-accelerated finite element method *Int. Conf. Modeling, Simulation, Optimization and Numerical Techniques (SMONT 2019)* (Paris: Atlantis)

Lou C, Nie L and Xu D 2011 Effect of excitation pulse width on thermoacoustic signal characteristics and the corresponding algorithm for optimization of imaging resolution *J. Appl. Phys.* **110** 275

Nie L, Ou Z, Yang S and Xing D 2010 Thermoacoustic molecular tomography with magnetic nanoparticle contrast agents for targeted tumor detection *Med. Phys.* **37** 4193–200

Paulsen K D and Jiang H 1996 Enhanced frequency-domain optical image reconstruction in tissues through total-variation minimization *App. Opt.* **35** 3447–58

Razansky D, Kellnberger S and Ntziachristos V 2010 Near-field radiofrequency thermoacoustic tomography with impulse excitation *Med. Phys.* **37** 4602–7

Rudin L I, Osher S and Fatemi E 1992 Nonlinear total variation based noise removal algorithm *Physica* D **60** 259–68

Shackelford R G 1962 Fresnel zone radiation patterns of microwave antennas *Master Degree Thesis* Georgia Institute of Technology

Stogryn A 1971 Equations for calculating the dielectric constant of saline water *IEEE Trans. Microw. Theory Tech.* **19** 733–6

van den Berg P M and Kleinmann R E 1995 A total variation enhanced modified gradient algorithm for profile reconstruction *Inverse Problems* **11** L5–L10

Wang B, Ma X, Liu S and Zhu X 2018 Efficient dictionary construction method for microwave induced thermoacoustic compressive sensing imaging *Appl. Phys. Lett.* **113** 053701

Wang X, Bauer D R, Vollin J L, Manzi D G and Xin H 2015 Impact of microwave pulses on thermoacoustic imaging applications *IEEE Antennas Wirel. Propag. Lett.* **11** 1634–7

Yao L and Jiang H 2011 Enhanced photoacoustic tomography using total variation minimization *Appl. Opt.* **50** 5031–41

Ye E, Ji Z, Ding W, Lou C, Yang S and Xing D 2016 Ultrashort microwave-pumped real-time thermoacoustic breast tumor imaging system *IEEE Trans. Med. Imaging* **35** 839–44

Yin C, Gao L and Liu K 2012 All solid state pulsed magnetron modulator based on MARX generator *Radar Sci. Technol.* **10** 223–26

Zheng Z, Huang L and Jiang H 2018 Label-free thermoacoustic imaging of human blood vessels *in vivo Appl. Phys. Lett.* **113** 253702

Zheng Z, Jiang Y C, Huang L, Zhao Y and Jiang H B 2020 An improved method for quantitative recovery of conductivity using tomographically measured thermoacoustic data *J. X-ray Sci. Technol.* **28** 137

Chapter 4

Transducer array-based TAT: 2D and 3D thermoacoustic imaging

In this chapter, we describe transducer-array-based thermoacoustic tomography (TAT) systems and demonstrate their ability for 2D and 3D thermoacoustic imaging of biological tissue.

4.1 Array-based TAT system and 2D imaging

Figures 4.1(a) and (b) present the photograph of an array-based TAT system. As shown in figure 4.1(a), a pulsed microwave generator is used to provide microwave pulses with a pulse width of 750 ns and a repetition rate of 1–1000 Hz. The thermoacoustic (TA) signals generated by the object are received by a transducer array with a frequency of 2.25 MHz or 8.5 MHz. Pre-amplifiers/amplifiers amplify the signals from the transducer array and deliver the amplified signals to the A/D boards which are controlled by the computer. The three key components of the system including the microwave generator, 128-element ultrasound transducer array and data acquisition system are discussed in detail in sections 4.1.1–4.1.3 below.

4.1.1 Microwave source

The microwave source is based on S-band magnetron oscillation, and has a center frequency of 3.0 GHz, a pulse width of 0.75 μs, peak a peak power of 70 kW, and a repetition rate of 1–1000 Hz. It is connected to an antenna by a coaxial line at the end of the waveguide. The microwave pulses propagating from the antenna port irradiate the object, and a 128-element ultrasound transducer array placed along the object receives the thermoacoustic signal from the object.

4.1.2 128-Element ultrasound transducer arrays

Figure 4.2(a) is the photograph of a flexible ultrasound transducer array. The flexible array consists of four segments, each of which has 32 elements with a center

doi:10.1088/978-0-7503-3163-0ch4

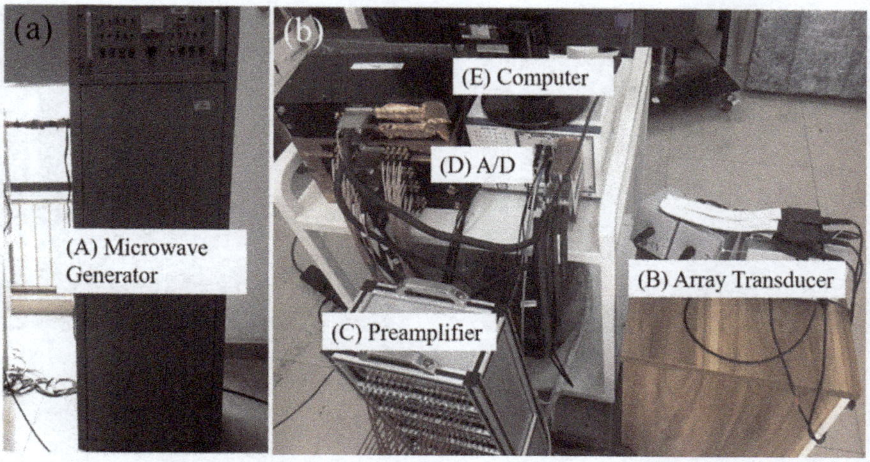

Figure 4.1. Photograph of the array-based TAT system. (a) Microwave generator. (b) The remaining components of the TAT system.

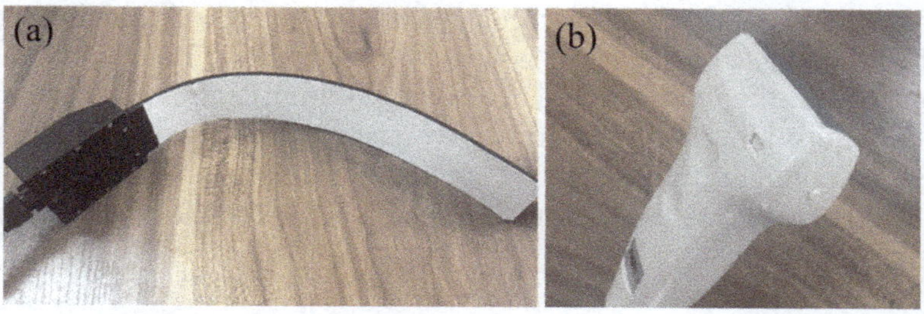

Figure 4.2. Photographs of the ultrasound transducer arrays. (a) The flexible ultrasound transducer array. (b) The linear ultrasound transducer array.

frequency of 2.25 MHz and a bandwidth of 70% for each element (2.25K3.0 × 10N-30CH P = 6.0, Japan probe, JAPAN). Figure 4.2(b) is the photograph of a linear ultrasound transducer array, which consists of 128 elements with a central frequency of 8.5 MHz for each element (SH7L38, SASET. Inc., China).

4.1.3 Control electronics and data acquisition

Adapted from Jiang (2014).

A 128-channel data acquisition system composed of eight pre-amplifiers, multiplexers and two data acquisition cards (NI5752, NI Inc. USA) is used to acquire the thermoacoustic signals. Each pre-amplifier/multiplexer includes 16 lMH6624 and 2 ADG1634 chips. Each pre-amplifier (i.e. AD8099) amplifies the signal with a gain of 26 dB. The whole system has 128 lMH6624 and 16 ADG1634 chips. Each NI5752 has 32 channels with a sample clock rate of up to 50 Ms s^{-1} and a 12-bit A/D converter. The system can acquire signals from 64 channels at one time. The computer sends out the scan enabling signals by the NI USB6501. All the channels will simultaneously convert the analog signals to digital data with user selected post

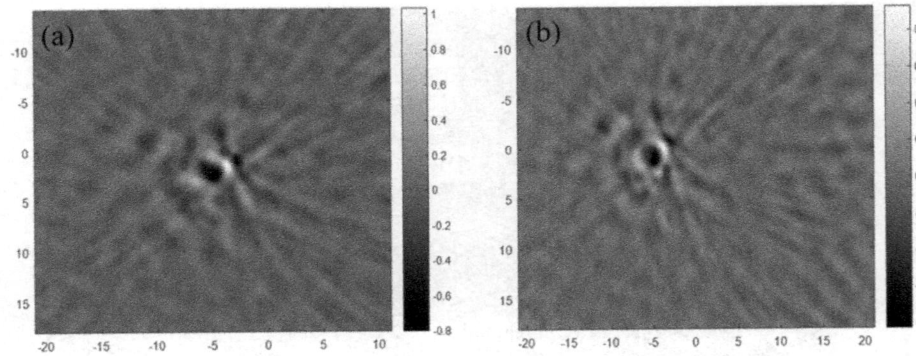

Figure 4.3. Thermoacoustic images of a 3 mm diameter saline-containing plastic tube. (a) Before calibration. (b) After calibration.

trigger delay and waveform length. Other programmable parameters include the sampling rate, trigger source, trigger rate, gain, DC offset, and low and high pass filters. Both boards feature user-selectable 12-bit resolution with up to 50 MB samples per second. With one board set as the master and the remaining set to slave mode, all the channels on the slave boards will start taking data upon receiving a trigger signal from the master board. Labview programming is used to control the entire data acquisition. The software is written to allow maximum flexibility for various system configurations. Pointers created during the data acquisition process are used to quickly access the thermoacoustic data. Data is then saved for off-line image reconstructions.

4.1.4 System evaluation and experimental studies

4.1.4.1 System calibration

The system calibration is primarily concerned with the calibration of the positioning and response of the multiple transducers in the system. We used a thermoacoustic point target centrally located to achieve the goal. In the calibration, the TA signal was measured by each transducer at all the locations along the circular path. Before calibration, we see that the signal from the point target arrived at each transducer at different times indicating positioning error. By adjusting the position of each transducer, we obtained the signals from the point target that arrived at the transducer at the same time point. Figure 4.3 shows the reconstructed image of one circular target before and after the calibration. We see that the calibration provides much improved image reconstruction in terms of the target shape and size.

4.1.4.2 Spatial resolution

To evaluate the system spatial resolution, we constructed a phantom consisting of two point targets (brass wires; 3 mm in diameter each). Figure 4.4(a) shows the reconstructed image of the two point targets, while figure 4.4(b) is the normalized profile of the reconstructed image along the red dot line shown in figure 4.4(a). From the profile, the half-width-at-half-maximum (AB) and the half-width-at-quarter-

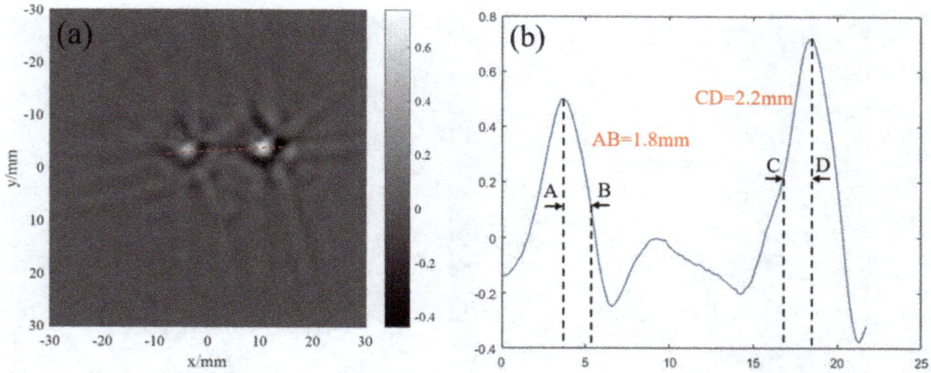

Figure 4.4. (a) Reconstructed image of two point targets. (b) Normalized profile of the reconstructed image along the red dot line shown in (a).

maximum (CD) were calculated to be 1.8 mm and 2.2 mm, respectively. Using the resolution criterion, the spatial resolution of the system was estimated to be AB + CD − target diameter = 1.8 + 2.2 − 3 = 1.0 mm.

4.1.4.3 Phantom evaluation

Phantom experiments were conducted to evaluate the 2D imaging ability of the array-based system. Here we show phantom results using the flexible transducer array as an example. Figures 4.5(a) and (b), respectively, show the recovered thermoacoustic image and the photograph of a triangular 2%-agar phantom, while figures 4.5(c) and (d) give the recovered thermoacoustic image and the photograph of a rectangle 2%-agar phantom with a 3 mm diameter saline-containing plastic tube embedded in the center of the agar phantom. The images obtained show that these targets with different sizes and shapes can be clearly detected using this array-based imaging system.

4.2 3D Imaging

For 3D imaging, while it is ideal to implement a 2D array of transducers, here we describe a 3D TAT system based on scanning a curved transducer array in *z*-direction. We demonstrate this TAT system using phantom experiments.

4.2.1 System description

Figure 4.6 depicts the experimental configuration of a 3D thermoacoustic imaging system. A microwave generator (peak power = 55 kW, frequency = 3.05 GHz, pulse duration tunable from 300 ns to 550 ns, and repetition rate = 100 Hz; Shichuan Huaweikang Medical Tech., Chengdu, China) is used to produce microwave pulses, which are delivered to the sample through a coaxial waveguide switch (aperture size: 50 × 30 mm^2) filled with transformer oil (relative permittivity = 2.3). A composite matching layer (relative permittivity = 12.5, loss tangent < 0.001, thickness = 7.2 mm) is attached to the waveguide to improve microwave transmission from the transformer oil into the sample immersed in deionized water. The sample generates TA

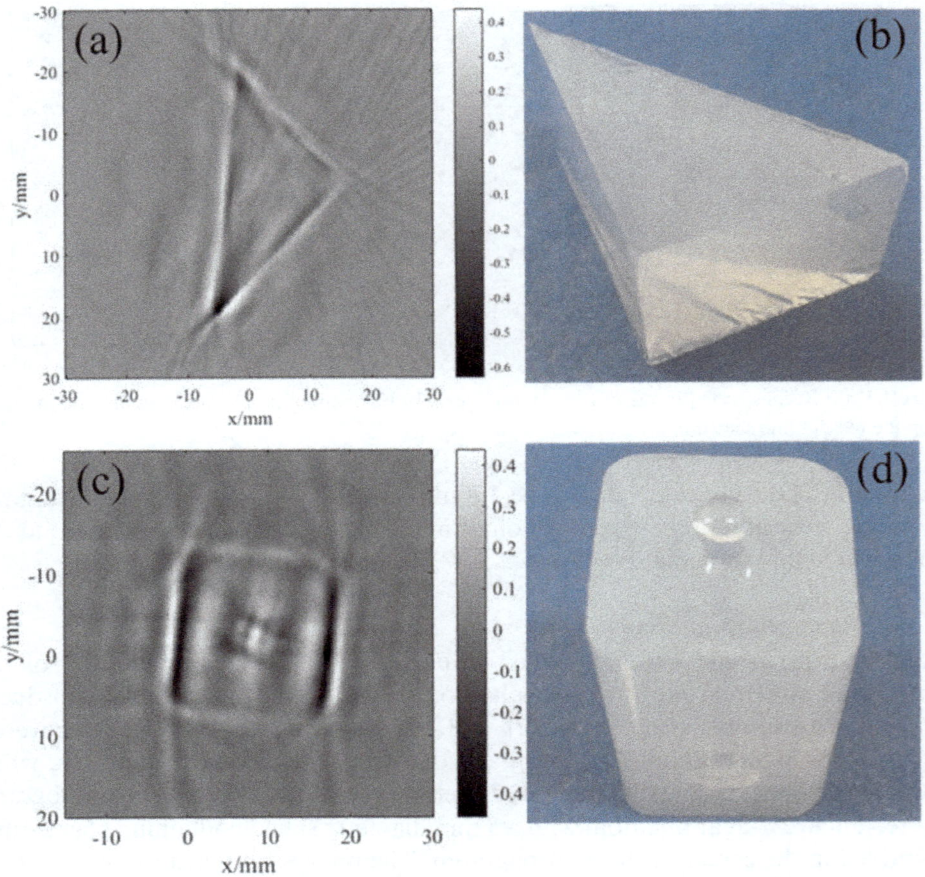

Figure 4.5. Cross-sectional TA images and photographs of differently-shaped 2%-agar phantoms.

signals when irradiated with a microwave pulse from the top. A 128-element cylindrically focused curved transducer array (central frequency: 5 MHz, bandwidth: 80%, Japan Probe Corporation, Yokohama, Japan) is used to acquire TA signals; the 128 elements are arranged in a half arc spanning 180° with a radius of 50 mm. A 128-channel pre-amplifier (60 dB) is used to amplify the signals, and the amplified TA signals are transferred to a 64-channel analog-to-digital system (5752B, National Instruments, Texas) at a sampling rate of 50 MS s^{-1} and 12-bit digital resolution after 2:1 multiplexing. One onboard computer (PXIe8840, National Instruments, Texas) controls the entire system and saves the acquired TA data.

For each transducer position, 1 s is needed to obtain the signals and a total of 84 s are needed to acquire a complete set of data for 3D imaging. Images are reconstructed with the delay-and-sum algorithm described in chapter 1. The 3D images are rendered with Amira (from Visage Imaging, Inc.).

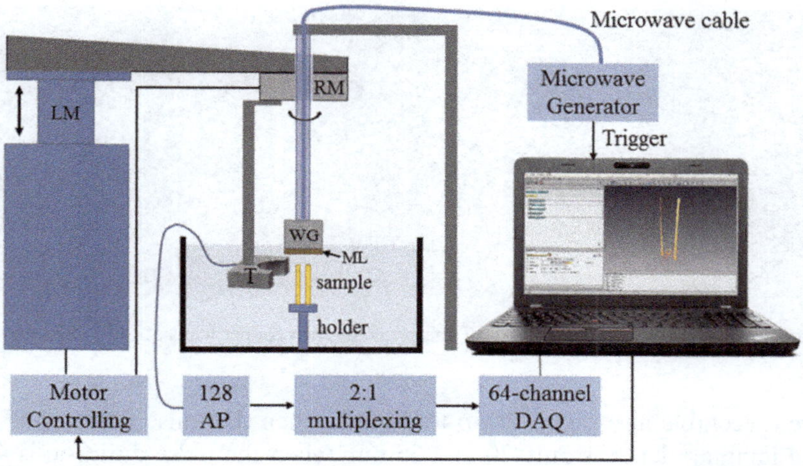

Figure 4.6. Experimental configuration of a 3D thermoacoustic imaging system. DAQ: data acquisition card, AP: amplifier, LM: linear translation step motor, RM: rotator step motor, WG: coaxial waveguide switch, ML: matching layer, T: ultrasonic transducer.

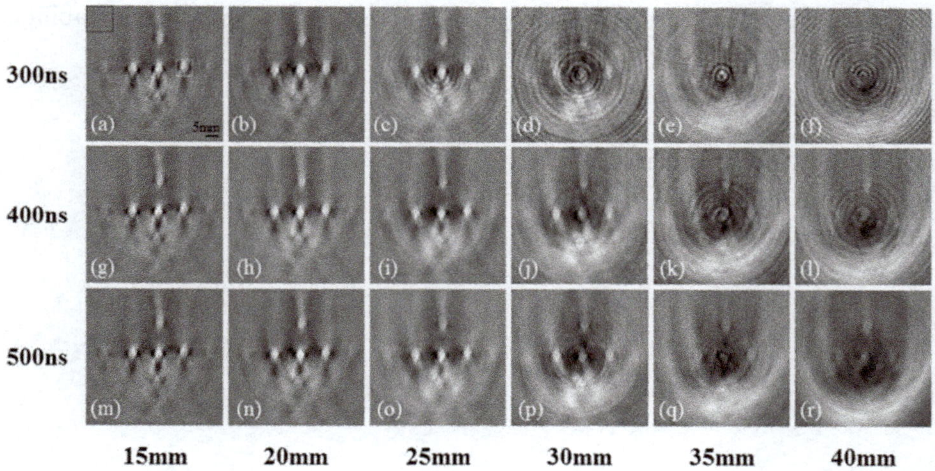

Figure 4.7. 2D TAT images of saline-containing plastic tubes placed at different depths when the pulse duration is 300 ns (a)–(f), 400 ns (g)–(l) and 500 ns (m)–(r), respectively.

4.2.2 Phantom experiments

Two different types of phantom experiments are conducted: one phantom consisting of an array of plastic tubes containing saline used to demonstrate the imaging depth with different widths of microwave pulse, and the other phantom consisting of two cooper wires to demonstrate the 3D imaging ability of the system. Figure 4.7 shows the reconstructed images of saline-containing plastic tubes placed at different depths when the width of the pulse is 300 ns (figures 4.7(a)–(f)), 400 ns (figures 4.7(g)–(l)) and 500 ns (figures 4.7(m)–(r)), respectively. From figure 4.7, we can see that the

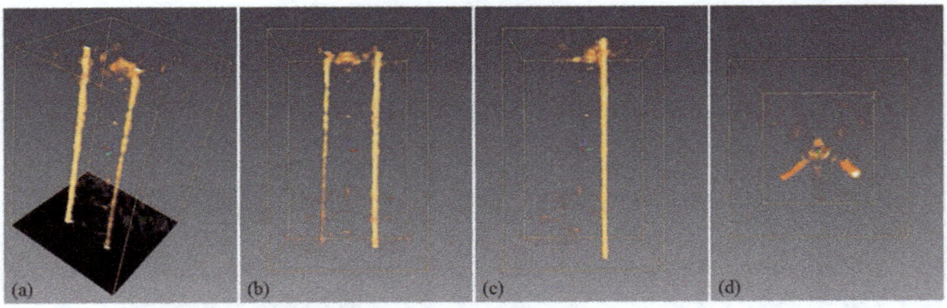

Figure 4.8. (a)–(d): Reconstructed 3D TAT images of the two cooper wires at four different views.

tubes are detectable at a depth of up to 40 mm when the pulse duration is 500 ns, while the imaging depth is only 30 and 25 mm when the pulse duration is 400 and 300 ns, respectively.

Figure 4.8 presents the reconstructed 3D images of the two copper wires at four different views. The reconstructed volume is 20 × 20 × 40 mm with a $0.1 \times 0.1 \times 0.5$ mm^3 voxel size. We see that the spatial distribution and the ends of the two cooper wires are clearly revealed, demonstrating the 3D imaging ability of this TAT system.

Reference

Jiang H 2014 Photoacoustic Imaging of Epilepsy *Report* W81XWH-09-1-0299

Chapter 5

High-resolution and multi-modal approaches

In this chapter, we describe some advanced thermoacoustic tomography (TAT) approaches, including high-resolution TAT and multi-modal approaches. Most TAT systems provide a spatial resolution of ~1 mm due to the limited microwave pulse widths (microseconds or sub-microseconds). This can be changed and a spatial resolution of ~100 μm or better can be reached when a microwave source that can generate pluses in the nanosecond range is used (Kellnberger *et al* 2011, Lou *et al* 2012, Razansky *et al* 2010).

When two or more different imaging modalities are physically combined appropriately, the combined system can take full advantage of different modalities to provide complementary information for most accurate clinical decision making. Here we present examples of combining TAT with several other modalities including photoacoustic tomography (PAT) and ultrasound (US) imaging to realize various TAT-based multi-modal approaches.

5.1 High-resolution TAT

As an example, we describe a high-resolution TAT method based on transmission lines that can generate tens of nanoseconds or even shorter microwave pulses (Omar *et al* 2012). For a transmission line pulse generator or pulser, one can scale the pulse duration by changing the length of the transmission line according to

$$\tau_{\text{pulse}} = \frac{2\ell_{\text{line}}}{c} \tag{5.1}$$

where $c = c_0/\sqrt{\varepsilon_r}$ is the phase velocity of the wave over the line, $c_0 = 3 \times 10^8\ \text{ms}^{-1}$ is the phase velocity of electromagnetic waves in free space, and ε_r is the relative permittivity of the dielectric separating the outer and the inner conductors. The amount of the stored energy in the transmission line pulser is given by the following equation:

doi:10.1088/978-0-7503-3163-0ch5

$$E_0 = \frac{1}{2}CV^2 \tag{5.2}$$

where E_0 is the amount of the stored energy, C is the capacitance of the line, and V is the charging voltage. We can see that the amount of the energy can be increased by either increasing the charging voltage, or by adding more and more lines in parallel, the increase in the stored energy in this case is proportional to the number of the lines, i.e. $E_{total} = N_{lines} \times E_0$.

As described in Omar *et al* (2012), a pulser could be constructed, which consisted of high-voltage coaxial lines (167–8556, Teledyne Reynolds), of three different lengths, i.e. 0.5, 1, and 2 m, having low attenuation at frequencies of up to 400 MHz. The output of the pulser was connected to a helically shaped energy coupling element, which was used to couple the electromagnetic energy to the object. A spark-gap capable of switching voltages of up to 36 kV within nanoseconds was used as a switch. The triggering of the spark-gap was realized via a function generator (DG-1022, Rigol Technologies Inc.), which feeds the trigger circuitry with triggering pulses at 10 Hz repetition rate. To maximize the delivered energy, three transmission lines were connected in parallel. A 30 kV high-voltage dc module (30C24- N125, HVProducts, USA) was used for charging the transmission lines. For TAT measurements, the object was placed onto a rotation stage (PRM1Z8, Thorlabs Inc.), which rotated the object over 360°. The generated thermoacoustic signals were detected by a cylindrically focused ultrasonic transducer (Model V382, Panametrics, Olympus NDT, USA). The detected signals were subsequently fed into a low-noise amplifier with 63 dB gain (AU-1291, MITEQ Inc., USA), and sampled by a digital oscilloscope (TDS3054B, Tektronix Inc., USA). Image reconstruction was performed using the delay-and-sum algorithm.

To show the imaging performance of the transmission-line-based TAT method, phantoms of three PVC tubes of 3.5 mm diameter were employed. In one phantom shown in figure 5.1(a) three tubes filled with saline (0.9% NaCl) were imaged where in a second phantom, figure 5.1(b), two tubes filled with saline and a third tube filled with deionized water were imaged instead. Strong signals were recorded coming from the highly conductive saline and were reconstructed as shown in figures 5.1(c) and (d). In comparison, the tube containing deionized water showed almost no contrast over the background. Figure 5.1(e) shows results from imaging a thin (50 μm diameter) metallic wire immersed in deionized water. The generated thermoacoustic signals were measured using a 15 MHz cylindrically focused transducer (Model V311, Panametrics, Olympus NDT, USA). Figure 5.1(e) gives a horizontal (H) and a vertical (V) profile through the reconstructed image of the wire shown in the inset. The achieved full-width-at-half-maximum (FWHM) of the reconstructed profile is ~60 μm. Upon deconvolution from a 50 μm rectangular function, corresponding to the wire's profile, one obtains an estimate of the FWHM of the point spread function of the system to be ~45 μm. This suggests that the use of the ultrashort pulses (i.e. nanoseconds) allows TAT imaging resolution limited only by the acoustic diffraction.

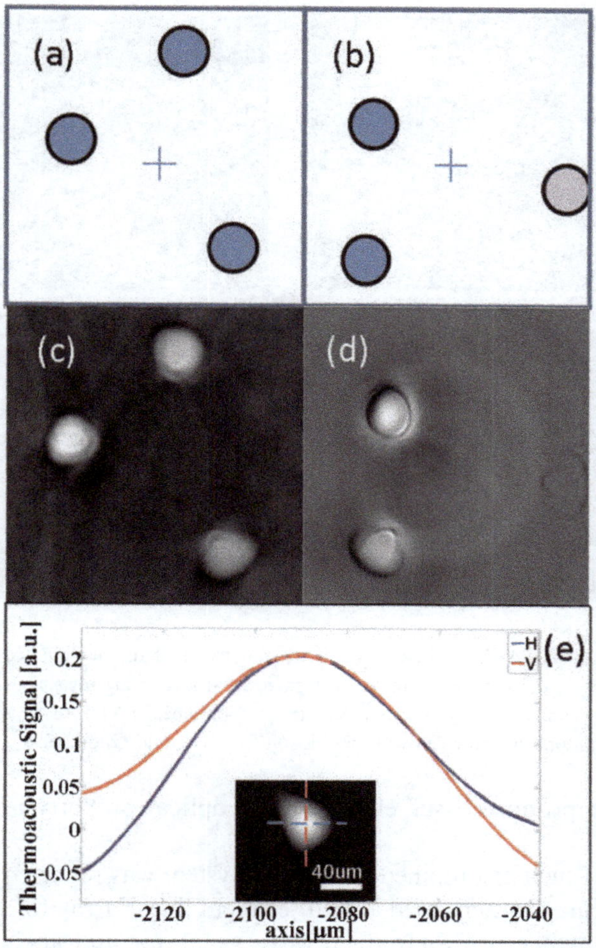

Figure 5.1. (a) Schematic pf Phantom 1 made of three plastic tubes containing saline and immersed in deionized water. (b) Schematic of Phantom 2 consisting of three plastic tubes, two tubes containing saline and one containing deionized water, also immersed in deionized water. (c) Reconstructed image of Phantom 1. (d) Reconstructed image of Phantom 2. (e) Cross-sectional profiles from imaging a 50 μm diameter metal wire. The inset shows a reconstruction of the wire. The line denoted by 'H' shows a horizontal profile through the reconstruction (horizontal line in inset) where the line denoted by 'V' depicts a corresponding vertical profile through the reconstruction (vertical dotted line). Adapted from Omar *et al* 2012, © John Wiley & Sons.

5.2 Multi-modal approaches—TAT/PAT

It is intuitive to combine thermoacoustic tomography (TAT) with photoacoustic tomography (PAT) for they have a similar contrast mechanism: TAT measures the ultrasonic waves induced by microwave pulses due to microwave absorption (tissue conductivity), while PAT detects the ultrasonic waves generated by laser pulses (tissue absorption). When TAT and PAT are combined, a common transducer or transducer array can be used to detect thermoacoustic (TA) or photoacoustic (PA) signals, and the same reconstruction algorithm can be used for TAT/PAT image

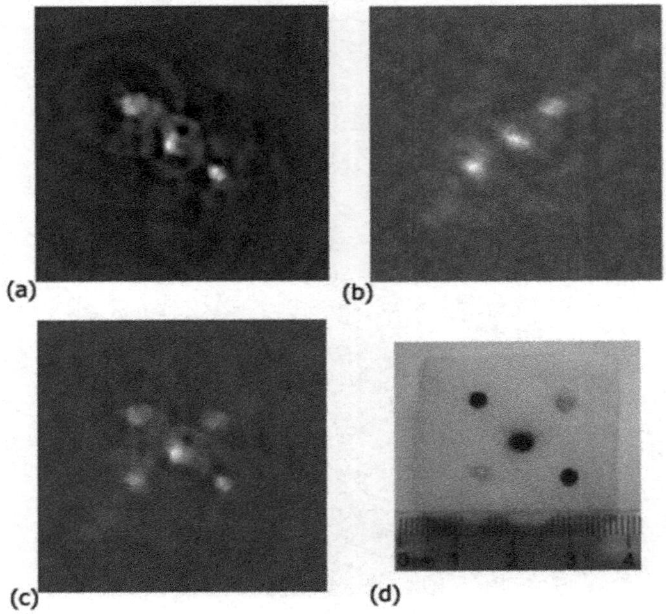

Figure 5.2. Cross-sectional TAT/PAT images of tissue mimicking phantom obtained from the TAT/PAT system. (a) PAT image of the sample where the two transparent targets are invisible. (b) TAT image of the sample where the two rubber targets are undetectable. (c) Combined TAT/PAT image of the sample. (d) Photograph of the phantom. Reproduced with permission from Nie and Guo (2009).

reconstruction to produce tissue electrical and optical property images in a single platform.

An example of such a combined TAT/PAT system was reported in Nie and Guo (2009). The combined system used a multi-element linear array for both TA and PA signal collection, while a 6 GHz microwave generator and an Nd:YAG laser at 532 nm were used for TA or PA excitation. The sample was placed on a rotary stage and immersed in a polyvinyl chloride tank filled with transformer oil. The system was tested using phantom experiments. The results are shown in figures 5.2(a)–(c), and 5.2(d) gives a photograph of the phantom where 5 targets (2 transparent agar, 1 agar mixed with India ink, and 2 black rubbers) were embedded in a piece of porcine fatty tissue. We see that PAT clearly detects the two black rubbers and the centrally located agar/ink target without seeing the two transparent targets, while TAT localizes the two transparent targets and the centrally located agar/ink target without recognizing the two rubber targets. Figure 5.2(c) presents the combined TAT/PAT image which provides all five targets.

5.3 Multi-modal approaches—TAT/US

While TAT can provide high-resolution tissue electrical property images, it often lacks certain tissue structural information. Combining ultrasound (US) imaging with TAT is one way to compensate this. In addition, TAT and US can share the common detection channel for ultrasound signal collection. We illustrate such a

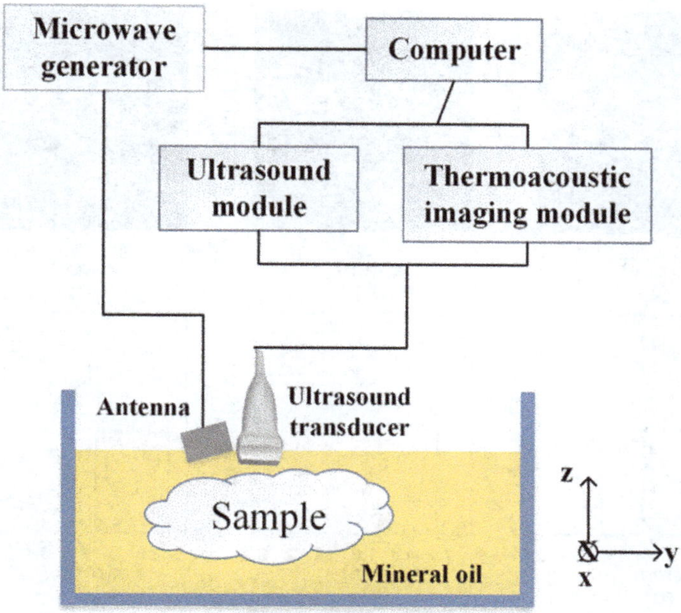

Figure 5.3. Schematic of a combined TAT/US system.

TAT/US combination using a linear transducer array as an example (see figure 5.3). In this TAT/US combined system, the ultrasound signal is generated, controlled and collected by the ultrasound module and then received by the linear array transducer. The thermoacoustic imaging module is used to amplify and collect the thermoacoustic signal through the linear array transducer. Moreover, the ultrasound and thermoacoustic imaging modules are switched on/off sequentially by a pinboard. In this way, the collected thermoacoustic and US images are rigorously registered.

Figure 5.4 shows the TAT (figure 5.4(a)) and US (figure 5.4(b)) images, and the fused TAT/US image (figure 5.4(c)) from a phantom experiment, in which three saline-containing tubes (3 mm in diameter each, see figure 5.4(g)) were imaged. Saline solution has been widely used as a phantom material for thermoacoustic imaging (Aliroteh and Arbabian 2018, Kellnberger *et al* 2011, Razansky *et al* 2010). Here, the saline-containing tubes were used to simulate the blood vessels. Microwave is an electrical signal, which can directly interfere with the signal generation in the ultrasonic transducer (Ding *et al* 2017). A distance of 10 mm was used to eliminate such an interference. The difference in the estimation of the target sizes for TAT and US is primarily due to the fact that TAT has lower resolution than US. Figures 5.4(d)–(f) show normalized profiles of these images along a cutting line through each target center (red line in figure 5.4(c)). From figures 5.4(d)–(f), we can calculate the full-width-at-half-maximum (FWHM) of each TA image profile and the distance between the two signal peaks in the US images as the diameter of targets, and find that the ultrasound images give a size of 2.79, 2.79 and 2.99 mm for the three targets, while the TA images provide a size of 3.36, 3.08 and 3.99 mm for the three targets. In addition, because of the use of a

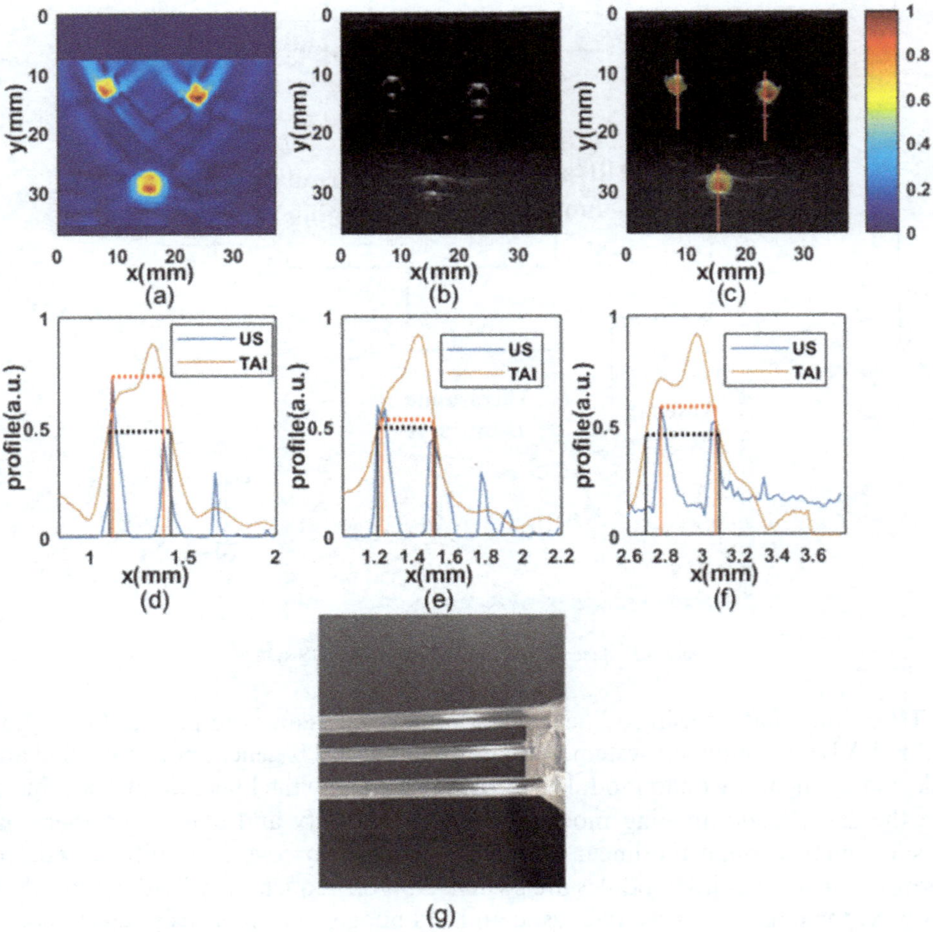

Figure 5.4. Phantom experiments for three saline-containing tubes. Thermoacoustic (a), ultrasound (b), and fused TAT/US images (c). (d)–(f) Image profiles along a cut line crossing the center of each target as indicated by red lines in (c), respectively. (g) is the photograph of the three saline-containing tubes. Color bar represents the relative TAT signal. Reprinted from Zheng *et al* (2018), with the permission of AIP Publishing.

transducer having a relatively high frequency, the boundary TA signal is stronger than the internal one. We see that all three targets are clearly detected in TAT and US with some artifacts for both TAT and US. These artifacts are almost removed when a threshold value is used (figure 5.4(c)). We also notice that the targets are shown as hollow ones in the ultrasound images, while they are shown as they actually are in the thermoacoustic images. (Adapted from Zheng *et al* 2018, with permission.)

References

Aliroteh M S and Arbabian A 2018 Microwave-induced thermoacoustic imaging of subcutaneous vasculature with near-field RF excitation *IEEE Trans. Microw. Theory Tech.* **66** 1–12

Ding W, Ji Z and Xing D 2017 Microwave-excited ultrasound and thermoacoustic dual imaging *Appl. Phys. Lett.* **110** 183701

Kellnberger S, Hajiaboli A, Razansky D and Ntziachristos V 2011 Near-field thermoacoustic tomography of small animals *Phys. Med. Biol.* **56** 3433–44

Lou C, Yang S, Ji Z, Chen Q and Xing D 2012 Ultrashort microwave-induced thermoacoustic imaging: a breakthrough in excitation efficiency and spatial resolution *Phys. Rev. Lett.* **109** 218101

Nie L and Guo H 2009 Thermoacoustic and photoacoustic imaging of biological tissue with different contrasts and properties *Proc. SPIE* **7280** 72801N

Omar M, Kellnberger S, Sergiadis G, Razansky D and Ntziachristos V 2012 Near-field thermoacoustic imaging with transmission line pulsers *Med. Phys.* **39** 4460–6

Razansky D, Kellnberger S and Ntziachristos V 2010 Near-field radiofrequency thermoacoustic tomography with impulse excitation *Med. Phys.* **37** 4602–7

Zheng Z, Huang L and Jiang H 2018 Label-free thermoacoustic imaging of human blood vessels *in vivo Appl. Phys. Lett.* **113** 253702

Chapter 6

Contrast agents-based molecular thermoacoustic imaging

Thus far our discussion on thermoacoustic tomography (TAT) principles has been based on endogenous contrast mostly due to water content and ion concentration. This native endogenous contrast may not be sufficient, and in many cases, the interactions of microwave with tissue are not disease specific. Thus, there is a significant role for exogenously administered contrast agents that have affinity for the disease site through biochemical interactions, providing not only highly sensitive but also disease-specific signals. The application of contrast agents is able to increase the sensitivity and specificity of TAT, rendering it a powerful molecular imaging tool. A targeted contrast agent can also be used for therapy in conjugation with drugs, and the double virtues of imaging and targeted therapy will then be possessed. In this chapter, we describe various exogenous contrast agents for thermoacoustic imaging including magnetic materials, and carbon nanomaterials among others.

6.1 Magnetic materials

6.1.1 Fe_3O_4/PANI and FA-Fe_3O_4/PANI

As described in Nie *et al* (2010), the synthesis of Fe_3O_4 cores follows a precipitation method. $FeCl_2{\cdot}4H_2O$ and $FeCl_3{\cdot}6H_2O$ are used as iron sources, while NaOH is used as a precipitator. Moreover, dodecylbenzene sulfonic acid sodium salt (NaDS) is used as a surfactant to prevent agglomeration among the nanoparticles. The precipitates are separated by magnetic decantation with acetone and pure water after cooling the suspension at room temperature. Coating of metallic oxide nanoparticles with PANIs is also straightforward. The Fe_3O_4/PANI nanoparticles with coreshell structure are synthesized using an *in situ* polymerization of aniline monomer in an aqueous solution, which contains well-dispersed Fe_3O_4 nanoparticles and NaDS as surfactant and dopant. Fe_3O_4 is the magnetic core, and these particles are polydisperse and some of these particles are agglomerated due to

doi:10.1088/978-0-7503-3163-0ch6

magnetodipole interactions among the particles. The Fe_3O_4 particles are almost spherical with diameters ranging from 10 to 30 nm. PANI is the aqueous and conducting shell, and can be easily conjugated to biomarkers. The Fe_3O_4/PANI particles are almost spherical with diameters ranging from 30 to 50 nm.

To synthesize Fe_3O_4/PANI with the ability to recognize tumor cells, folate receptor (FR) as a tumor marker is selected. FR is a highly selective tumor receptor overexpressed in cancer cell membranes. Folic acid (FA) serves as a tumor-homing molecule that can guide Fe_3O_4/PANI into FR-overexpressed tumor cells. Specifically, FA (1 mg ml^{-1}) is dissolved in dimethyl sulfoxide (DMSO) and activated by 1-ethyl-3-(3-(dimethylamino)-propyl) carbodiimide (EDC)/*N*-hydroxysulfonosuccinimide (NHS) to afford FA-NHS (molar ratio, FA:EDC:NHS = 1:1:1). Fe_3O_4/PANI is mixed with FA-NHS and incubated without light exposure for 12 h. The resulting product, FA-Fe_3O_4/PANI, is dialyzed against phosphate-buffered saline (PBS) using 1000 Da filter (Millipore) to remove free FA, EDC/NHS, and FA-NHS.

In vivo experiments are used to demonstrate the ability of enhancing TAT using Fe_3O_4/PANI and FA-Fe_3O_4/PANI. TAT images of *in vivo* mouse tail are obtained without (figure 6.1(a)) and with (figure 6.1(b)) Fe_3O_4/PANI nanoparticles. The experiments are conducted using a TAT system shown in figure 6.1(c) where the TA signal receiving plane of the linear transducer array (2.5 MHz each element) is vertical to the microwave illumination direction (6 GHz). We see that the TAT image after the administration of the nanoparticles shows clearly increased signal in the target (blood vessels) (figure 6.1(b)) compared to that without the use of the nanoparticles (figure 6.1(a)).

Figure 6.2 gives the TAT images of a tumor-bearing mouse before (figure 6.2(a) and (d)) and after (figure 6.2(b) and (e)) the injection of Fe_3O_4/PANI (figure 6.2(b)) or FA-Fe_3O_4/PANI (figure 6.2(e)). We note that the tumor signal (dashed ellipses) after the injection of nanoparticles is significantly increased, especially after the

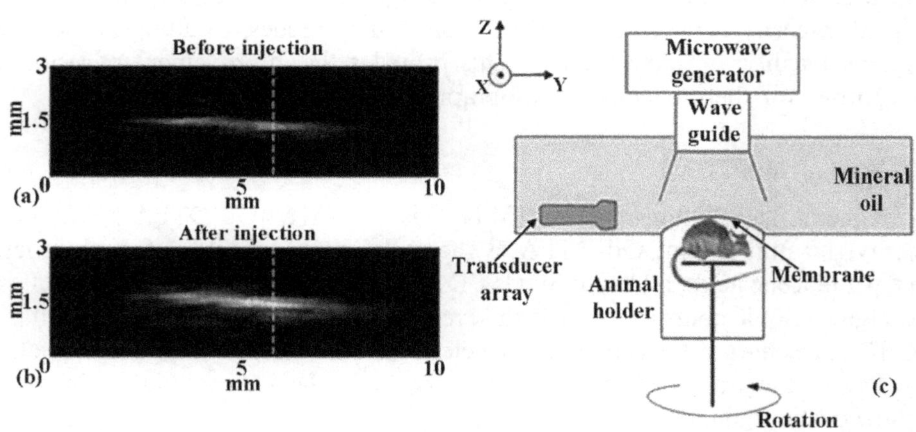

Figure 6.1. *In vivo* TAT images of a mouse tail before (a) and after (b) intravenous injection of Fe_3O_4/PANI. (c) Schematic of the TAT system used for the *in vivo* demonstration. Reproduced with permission from Nie *et al* (2010), © John Wiley & Sons..

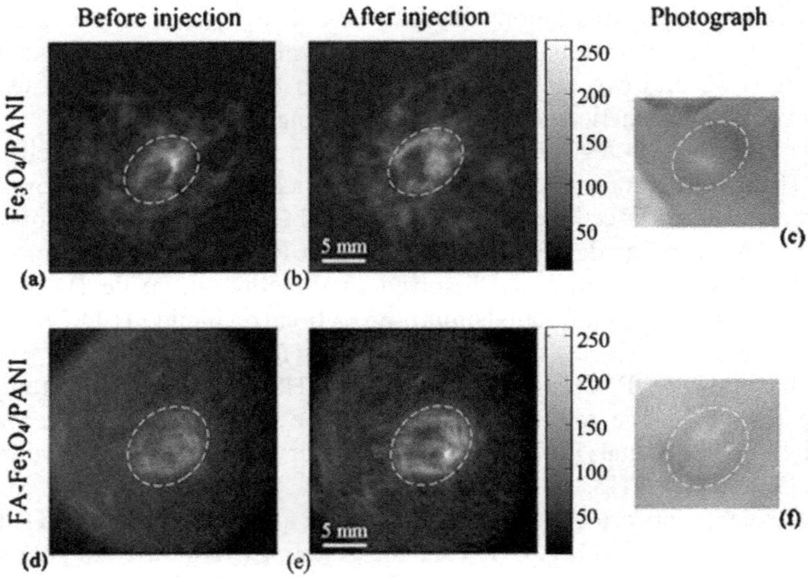

Figure 6.2. *In vivo* TAT images of a tumor-bearing mouse before (a), (d) and after (b), (e) the injection of Fe_3O_4/PANI (b) or FA-Fe_3O_4/PANI (e). (c) and (f) Photographs of the tumor area on the mouse back. Reproduced with permission from Nie *et al* (2010), © John Wiley & Sons.

injection of FA-Fe_3O_4/PANI (figure 6.2(e) versus (d)), while the endogenous contrast of the tumor provides detectable TA signal for both cases (figure 6.2(a) and (d)).

Other variations of Fe_3O_4 particles such as dextran-coated Fe_3O_4 can also be used as a contrast agent for enhanced TAT (Qin *et al* 2011). Dextran-coated Fe_3O_4 magnetic nanoparticles administered intravenously are phagocytosed by resident Kupffer cells in normal reticuloendothelial system (RES) within the liver, but are not retained in tumor tissue. Hence, there exists a significant difference in thermoacoustic signal intensity between normal RES and tumor tissues, resulting in increased tumor conspicuity and detectability. This provides the improvement of lesion-to-liver contrast for thermoacoustic tomography.

6.1.2 NMG_2[Gd(DTPA)]

Paramagnetic gadolinium chelate (Magnevist®, NMG_2[Gd(DTPA)]: NMG = *N*-methylglucammonium; Gd-DTPA = the gadolinium complex of diethylenetriamine pentaacetic acid), a United States FDA approved contrast agent for MRI, is a paramagnetic ionic contrast agent with seven unpaired electrons in the 4f orbital of the Gd^{3+}. The charged ions and unpaired electrons can interact with microwave field and convert the absorbed microwave energy into heat, resulting in increased thermoacoustic signal.

To show that NMG_2[Gd(DTPA)] can be used as a contrast agent for TAT, a TA signal of 0.5M NMG_2[Gd(DTPA)] is measured and compared with that of water, blood, muscle, and fat using a TAT system 6 GHz (Qin *et al* 2012). The TA signals

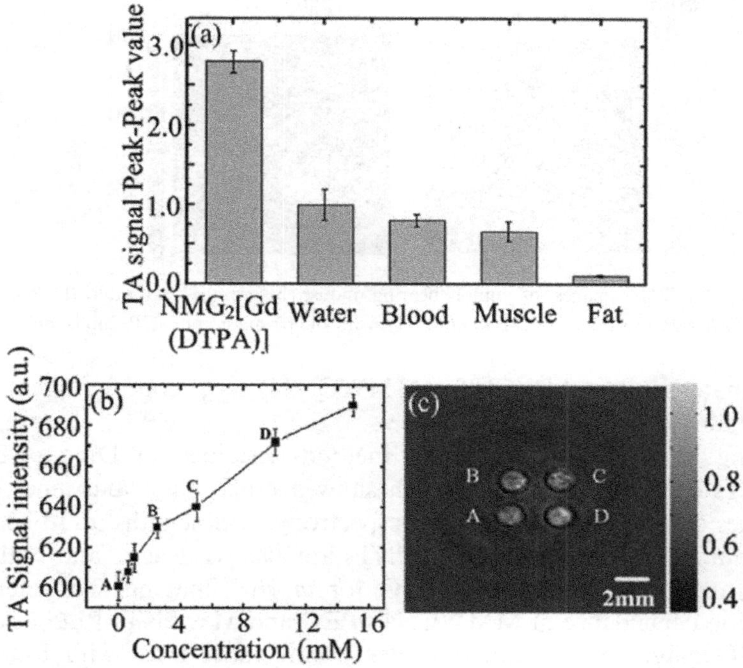

Figure 6.3. (a) TA signals of 0.5M $NMG_2[Gd(DTPA)]$ solution, water, blood, muscle and fat. (b) TA signals of $NMG_2[Gd(DTPA)]$ at different concentrations. (c) TAT images of $NMG_2[Gd(DTPA)]$ of four 1.8 mm diameter plastic tubes containing different concentrations in paraffin. A: water, B: 2.5 mM $NMG_2[Gd(DTPA)]$, C: 5 mM $NMG_2[Gd(DTPA)]$, D: 10 mM $NMG_2[Gd(DTPA)]$. Reprinted from Qin *et al* (2012), with the permission of AIP Publishing.

generated by $NMG_2[Gd(DTPA)]$ solution, water, blood, muscle, and fat are given in figure 6.3(a) where we see that the TA signal of $NMG_2[Gd(DTPA)]$ solution is considerably stronger than that of water, blood, muscle or fat. TA signals of $NMG_2[Gd(DTPA)]$ at different concentrations are also measured (figure 6.3(b)). We note that the TA signal of $NMG_2[Gd(DTPA)]$ increases with increased particle concentration. Figure 6.3(c) shows the TAT images of four 1.8 mm diameter plastic tubes having different concentrations of $NMG_2[Gd(DTPA)]$ solution embedded in paraffin. From figure 6.3(c), the different contrasts for these four tubes are revealed.

In vivo TAT images of tumor-bearing mouse before and after the injection of $NMG_2[Gd(DTPA)]$ are shown in figure 6.4. A clear increase in TA signal in the tumor especially in the tumor boundary after the injection of the particles is seen (figure 6.4(b)) compared to that before the injection of the particles (figure 6.4(a)).

6.2 Carbon nanomaterials

Various carbon materials can be used as contrast agents for TAT, including carbon nanoparticles, single-walled carbon nanotubes (SWCNTs), multi-walled carbon nanotubes (MWCNTs), and graphene nanoribbons and nanoplatelets (Gao *et al* 2017, Mashal *et al* 2010). Here we present an example using MWCNTs, specifically,

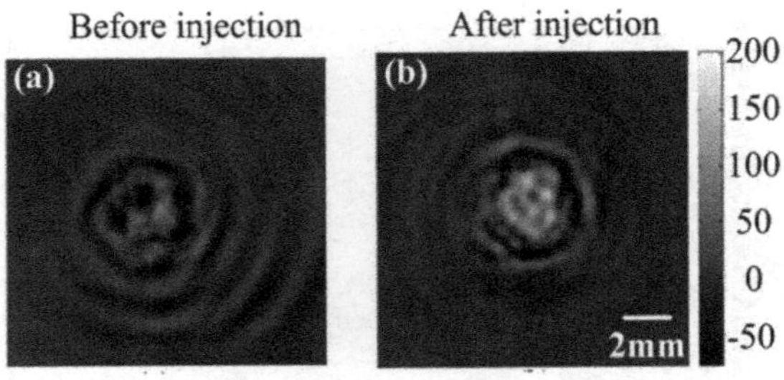

Figure 6.4. *In vivo* TAT images of tumor bearing mouse before (a) and after (b) the injection of NMG_2[Gd(DTPA)]. Reprinted from Qin *et al* (2012), with the permission of AIP Publishing.

magnetic material-filled MWCNTs (MMWCNTs) as a contrast agent for TAT (Ding *et al* 2016).

Following an *in situ* solvothermal method described in Ding *et al* (2016), MMWCNTs can be synthesized, which show average outer and inner diameters in the ranges of 30–40 and 10–20 nm, respectively, with lengths up to between 500 and 1500 nm. As a comparison, MWCNTs are also used here, and both types of nanotubes are functionalized with PEG for *in vivo* imaging. To determine the concentration dependence of MMWCNTs-PEG and MWCNTs-PEG as a contrast agent, TAT images of 0.7 mm diameter plastic tubes filled with four different concentrations (0.10, 0.25, 0.5, and 0.75 mg ml^{-1}) of CNTs are obtained (figure 6.5(a)). We note that the contrast of the tubes increases with increased concentration of MMWCNTs-PEG or MWCNTs-PEG. In particular, the contrast of the tubes filled with MMWCNTs-PEG is clearly larger than MWCNTs-PEG-containing tubes at the same concentration. In addition, T2 MR images of MMWCNTs-PEG and MWCNTs-PEG at 0.5 mg ml^{-1} concentration are provided (figure 6.5(b) (left)). Quantitative TA signals extracted from figure 6.5(a) are shown in figure 6.5(b) (left) where again we see that MMWCNTs offer a larger increase in TA signal compared to MWCNTs at a common concentration.

In vivo imaging of a breast tumor-bearing mouse is demonstrated using MMWCNTs-PEG tagged with folic acid (FA). MWCNTs-PEG-FA and MMWCNTs-PEG-FA (200 μL, 0.10 mg ml^{-1}) are injected through the mouse's tail-vein. TAT and MRI are performed before and after the injection of the nanotubes (figure 6.6(a)–(h)). We immediately note that the mouse injected with MMWCNTs-PEG-FA (figure 6.6(h)) shows significantly larger TA signal than that injected with MWCNTs-PEG-FA (figure 6.6(f)). The T2 intensity and TA signal profiles in the tumor are given in figure 6.6(i) and (j), respectively. We see that MMWCNTs-PEG-FA provides a significantly larger TA contrast enhancement compared to MWCNTs-PEG-FA.

6.3 Other materials

TAT contrast agents described in sections 6.1 and 6.2 are mostly based on nanomaterials. In fact, other non-nanomaterials such as air-filled microbubbles and saline have the potential to become effective contrast agents for enhanced TAT.

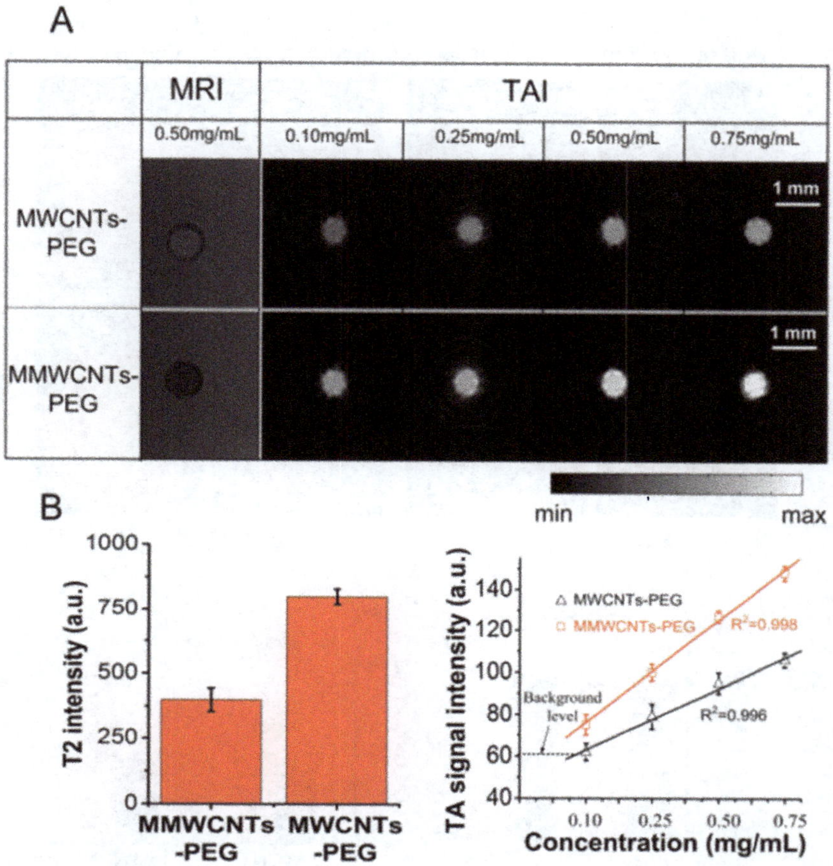

Figure 6.5. Concentration dependence of MMWCNTs-PEG and MWCNTs-PEG. (A) TAT images of MWCNTs-PEG and MMWCNTs-PEG at different concentrations and T2-weighted MR image of MWCNTs-PEG and MMWCNTs-PEG at 0.50 mg ml^{-1}. (B) Quantified T2-weighted MR signal intensity and quantification of TA signals. Note that TAI = TAT. Reprinted from Ding *et al* (2016), Copyright 2016, with permission from Elsevier.

It has been shown that the interstitial infusion of microbubbles to a tumor site, for example, will create a smaller thermoacoustic response compared to the pre-contrast-agent response, thereby enhancing sensitivity through the use of differential imaging techniques (Mashal *et al* 2009). In this case, the relative permittivity and conductivity of tissue decrease with increased microbubble concentration. A recent study shows that saline can provide strong contrast at physiologically acceptable concentrations, due to its ability to form strong electrolytes and increase ionic conductivity (Ogunlade and Beard 2014). For both microbubbles and saline, however, *in vivo* experiments remain to be performed to show the true potential of these materials as an effective contrast agent for TAT.

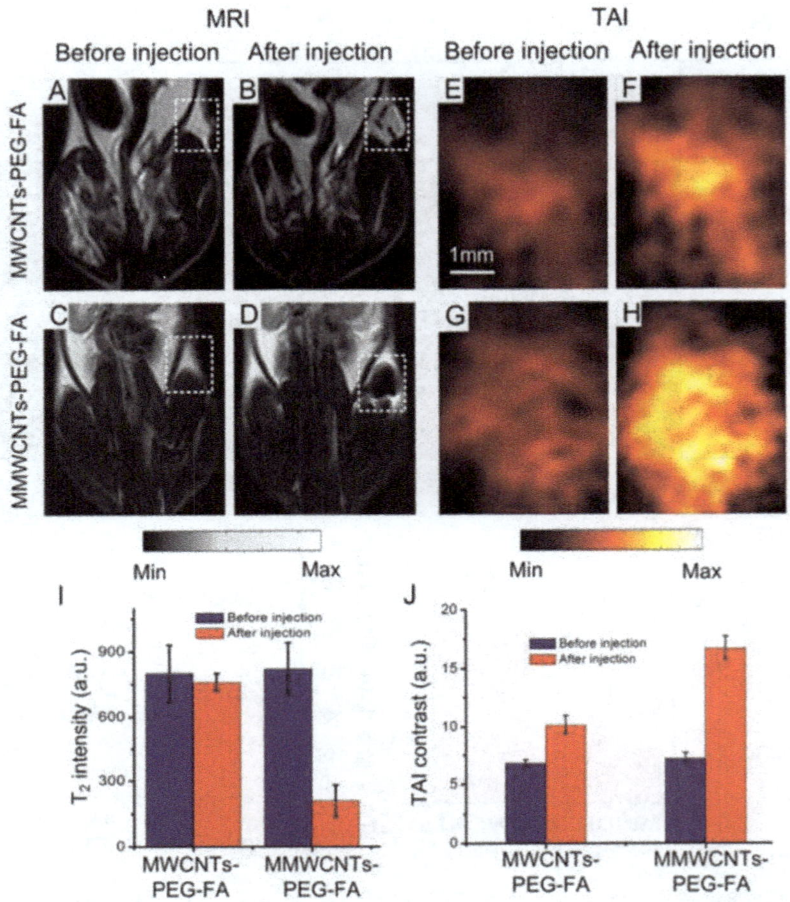

Figure 6.6. *In vivo* MRI and TAT imaging of a tumor-bearing mouse. (A)–(D) MRI images (TE = 79.6 ms; TR = 4460 ms) of one slice through the tumor. (E)–(H) TAT images of one slice through the tumor. (I) Quantification of the T2-weighted MR signals intensity of the tumors. (J) The TA signal of the tumors. Note that TAI = TAT. Reprinted from Ding *et al* (2016), Copyright 2016, with permission from Elsevier.

References

Ding W, Lou C, Qiu J, Zhao Z, Zhou Q, Liang M, Yang S, Ji Z and Xing D 2016 Targeted Fe-filled carbon nanotube as a multifunctional contrast agent for thermoacoustic and magnetic resonance imaging of tumor in living mice *Nanomed.-Nanotechnol* **12** 235–44

Gao F, Kishor R, Feng X, Liu S, Ding R, Zhang R and Zheng Y 2017 An analytical study of photoacoustic and thermoacoustic generation efficiency towards contrast agent and film design optimization *Photoacoustics* **7** 1–11

Mashal A, Booske J H and Hagness S C 2009 Toward contrast-enhanced microwave-induced thermoacoustic imaging of breast cancer: an experimental study of the effects of micro-bubbles on simple thermoacoustic targets *Phys. Med. Biol.* **54** 641–50

Mashal A, Sitharaman B, Li X, Avti P K, Sahakian A V, Booske J H and Hagness S C 2010 Toward carbon-nanotube-based theranostic agents for microwave detection and treatment of breast cancer: enhanced dielectric and heating response of tissue-mimicking materials *IEEE T. Bio. Med. Eng.* **57** 1831–4

Nie L, Ou Z, Yang S and Xing D 2010 Thermoacoustic molecular tomography with magnetic nanoparticle contrast agents for targeted tumor detection *Med. Phys.* **37** 4193–200

Ogunlade O and Beard P 2014 Electric and magnetic properties of contrast agents for thermoacoustic imaging *Phot. Plus Ultrasound: Imag. Sens.* **8943** 89432V

Qin H, Xu D and Yang S 2011 Dextran-coated Fe_3O_4 magnetic nanoparticles as a contrast agent in thermoacoustic tomography for hepatocellular carcinoma detection *J. Phys. Conf. Ser.* **277** 012028

Qin H, Yang S and Xing D 2012 Microwave-induced thermoacoustic computed tomography with a clinical contrast agent of NMG_2[Gd(DTPA)] *Appl. Phys. Lett.* **100** 033701

Chapter 7

Clinical applications and animal studies

In this chapter, we discuss the applications of thermoacoustic tomography (TAT) to several clinically significant areas and demonstrate its validity in humans and in animals. As we see from the contents presented below, the unique high contrast in tissue conductivity (and dielectric property) coupled with the high spatial and large depth resolutions render TAT an excellent modality for various tissue types/organ sites including the brain, breast, joints, thyroid, liver and vasculatures.

7.1 Joint imaging

Arthritis is the leading cause of disability in the population amongst over 50-year-olds and is associated with activity limitation, employment obstacles, reduced quality of life and increased medical costs. However, diagnosis of joint diseases (including arthritis and trauma) is a complex problem because of the structural complexity and diversity of disorders (Balakrishnan *et al* 2014, Erickson *et al* 1989, Wieschhoff *et al* 2016).

Current clinical diagnostic techniques for evaluating joint diseases, have strengths and weaknesses (Brown 2009, Chan *et al* 1991, Smith and Moran 2006, Vasanth *et al* 2010). X-ray and computed tomography (CT) have the advantage of excellent visualization of hard tissues, and are primarily used for bony abnormalities. X-ray and CT, however, are insensitive to changes in soft tissues include cartilage and synovium. In addition, they use ionizing radiation. Ultrasound (US) is portable, low in cost, capable of real-time assessment, and non-ionizing, and performs better than x-ray in imaging soft tissues. US is used to evaluate thickness of articular cavity, and allows visualization of pannus and edema. However, US is less suitable for minor lesions in early arthritis and cannot display the abnormalities in the subchondral bone due to its inability to penetrate the bone. Magnetic resonance imaging (MRI) represents a powerful modality for evaluating joint abnormalities include soft tissues and bone, because of its high sensitivity, specificity, and accuracy, particularly when a surface coil or contrast agent is used. However, MRI is expensive and may not be suitable for long-term, routine monitoring of joint diseases.

For joint diseases, the knee joint and interphalangeal joints are damaged earliest or most severely (Bijlsma *et al* 2011, Delport 2015, Smith and Moran 2006, Vohra *et al* 2011). Abnormal use or chronic use of the knee joint when doing exercises and manual labor involving twist and stretch can easily cause acute injuries and chronic diseases ranging from the trivial to the devastating. Two clinical phenotypes predominate in arthritis: osteoarthritis (OA) and rheumatoid arthritis (RA) (Bolen *et al* 2005, Hart and Spector 2000). Knee and hip OA bear most responsibility for the burden of OA; hand OA may be an important indicator of a systemic tendency to OA, among which the distal and proximal interphalangeal joints (DIP and PIP) are most frequently affected (Balakrishnan *et al* 2014, Hochberg 1991, Sarzi-Puttini *et al* 2005, Sun *et al* 2011). Also, as a symmetric polyarticular arthritis, RA primarily affects the small diarthrodial joints of the hands and feet (Alamanos and Drosos 2005, Firestein 2003, Marrelli *et al* 2011, Van Es *et al* 2015). Compared with hand OA, hand RA is distributed to the metacarpophalangeal joint and PIP. Distal interphalangeal joints are seldom involved (Altman 1990).

Here, we first present an animal study in thermoacoustic imaging of rabbit knee joints (Reprinted, with permission, from Chi *et al* 2016). We then evaluate the performance of TAT in imaging healthy human joints (Reprinted, with permission, from Chi *et al* 2019). Finally, we show the ability of TAT in detecting rheumatoid arthritis in the finger joints.

7.1.1 Rabbit knee joints

7.1.1.1 Animal model

Reprinted, with permission from Wiley, from Chi *et al* (2016).

Adult New Zealand male rabbits (average weight = 2 kg) were chosen for this study. In a TAI experiment, a rabbit was placed in a holder to maintain a genuflex position after being injected with pentobarbital through its ear margin intravenous (30 mg kg^{-1}). The holder and the rabbit were then positioned under the horn antenna of the TAI system for signal acquisition and image reconstruction. After the experiment, the imaged knee joint was dissected and photographed. Identical procedures were performed for several rabbits ($n = 4$). Finally, detailed comparative analyses between TAI images and anatomical pictures of the knee joint were conducted.

7.1.1.2 Imaging system

The experimental system used for *in vivo* rabbit knee joints is schematically shown in figure 7.1. The rabbit to be imaged was placed in a plastic holder to keep its knee joint under the horn antenna; both the holder and rabbit body (excluding the head) were immersed in an organic glass tank filled with mineral oil. The transducer received the acoustic signals at 130 positions (within 260°) via a step motor rotating the receiver around the knee joint. The knee joint was fixed in a genuflex position, the most common posture when the rabbit was free. In order to reduce the burden of

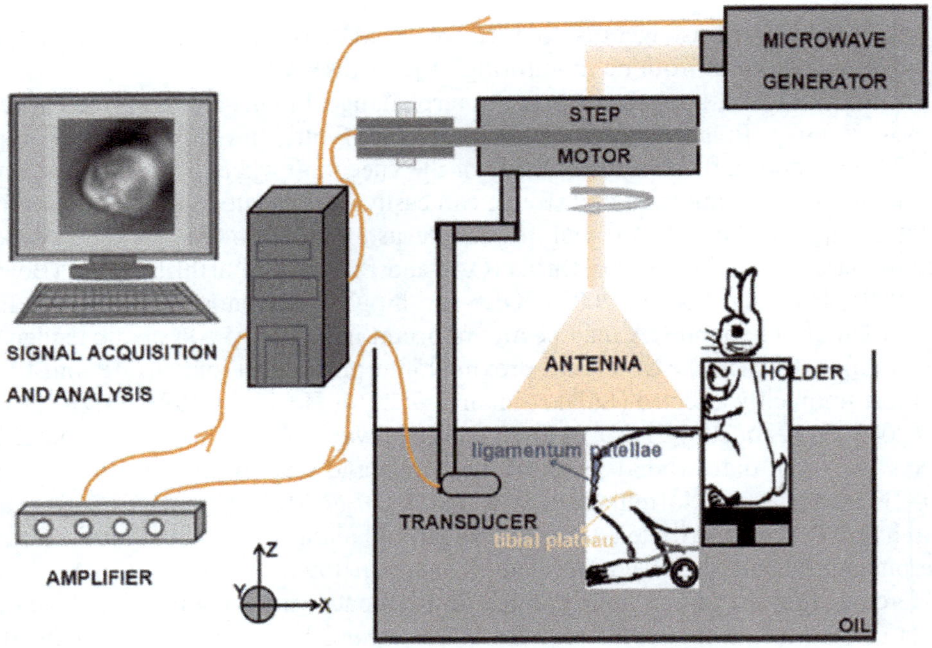

Figure 7.1. Schematic of the TAT system for imaging of rabbit knee joints. Reproduced from Chi *et al* (2016), © John Wiley & Sons.

the knee joint and unnecessary contact between the rabbit body and oil, the rabbit was kept in a sitting position in the holder. In such position, axial images of the joint were acquired and the axial anatomy (i.e. photograph of *ex vivo* joint tissues after the TAT scanning) was used for comparison (Reicher *et al* 1985).

It is necessary to indicate the advantages and disadvantages associated with the rabbit in a genuflex position in the experiment. With this design, the pulsed microwave could be delivered directly to the knee joint without passing through other parts of the body, as shown in figure 7.1. While the ultrasound signal from the anterior portions of the knee joint could be efficiently detected, the detection of the signal produced by the posterior portions of the knee joint was affected. The influence included two aspects. First, the thigh and calf tissues were pressed together and positioned right behind the knee joint. Second, the holder in the oil allowed the transducer to rotate only 260°, and the missing 100° just covered the posteromedial and posterior portions of the knee.

7.1.1.3 Image reconstruction

Several signal processing methods were applied before the thermoacoustic (TA) data were used for image reconstruction using the delay-and-sum method (Hoelen and de Mul 2000).

The original TA data were also processed in both time- and frequency-domain to remove system noises. In time-domain, there were impulse signals having quite short pulse widths and far higher amplitudes than that of the TA signals produced by the tissues (figure 7.2(a)). These impulse noises were produced when the electrical

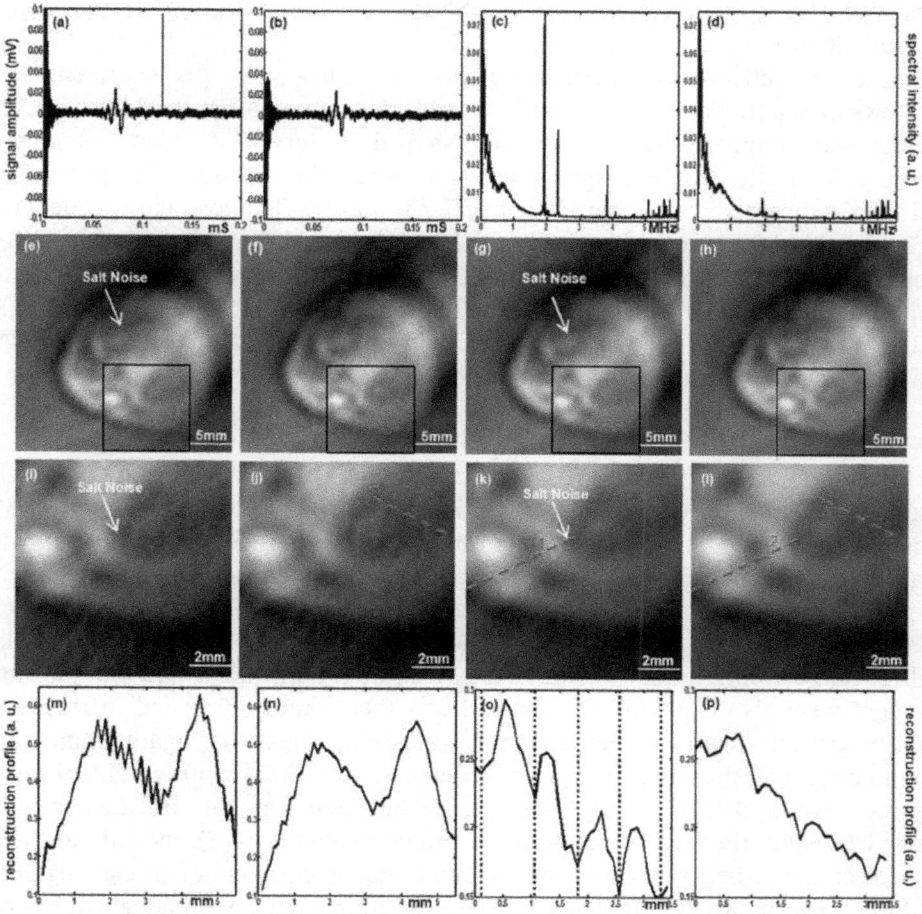

Figure 7.2. Signal processing. Signal waveforms in time-domain ((a) and (b)) and frequency-domain ((c) and (d)) from one detector position: original ((a) and (c)) and threshold or band-stop processed ((b) and (d)). Reconstructed TAT images without signal processing (e), and with threshold method (f), filtering (g), and both threshold and filtering processing (h). Enlarged images ((i)–(l)) for areas indicated by black squares in (e)–(h), respectively. Recovered profiles ((m)–(p)): plotted along dashed lines ((1)–(4)) from the images shown in figures 7.2(j)–(l), respectively. Reproduced from Chi *et al* (2016), © John Wiley & Sons.

switches in the system changed state, and by electromagnetic interference as well. These noises were removed by setting a suitable threshold with a value lower than the noise but higher than the true signal (figure 7.2(b)). Similar phenomena could also be seen in the frequency spectra (figure 7.2(c)). In this case, some band-stop filters were used to filter out the noises, as shown in figure 7.2(d). Time-domain impulse noisy signals existed in the form of white spots in the TAT images, namely, salt noise as shown in figure 7.2(e) and these spots were removed, as shown in figure 7.2(f). Comparing between figures 7.2(e) and (g), the reconstructed image became clearer only after the filtering. Both the signal processing methods effectively improved the signal-to-noise ratio (SNR) of the resulting TAT images (figure 7.2(h)).

In order to better show the denoising effect, in figures 7.2(i)–(l), we present close-up views of selected areas indicated by the black squares in figures 7.2(e)–(h). The profile was improved from serration-shaped (figure 7.2(m)) to smoothed (figure 7.2(n)) after impulse signals were removed. The salt noise in figures 7.2(i) and (k) disappeared, as shown in figures 7.2(j) and (l). The average wavelength λ used was about 0.81 mm and $f = v/\lambda = 1.85$ MHz ($v = 1.5$ mm/μs was the average acoustic velocity), which matched well with the frequency at the maximum amplitude noise shown in figure 7.2(c). The puddle-like artifacts in figures 7.2(i) and (j) were reduced, as shown in figures 7.2(k) and (l). Overall, the quality of TAT images was improved after the signal processing.

7.1.1.4 Results and discussion

As the anatomical pictures of the knee joint were used as the 'gold' standard in this study, let us first describe the relative positions of several major tissues. Figure 7.3(a) shows the picture of the knee joint (without the skin) when the knee was in the imaging position (see figure 7.1). In this case, the ligamentum patellae was almost perpendicular to the imaging plane. Figure 7.3(b) gives the picture after the patella was stripped off from the femur and the contact between the ligamentum patellae and the surrounding tissues was removed. We noted that the fat pad and the small ligament were also exposed. The fat pad was then bluntly dissected to reveal the anterior cruciate ligament, the posterior cruciate ligament, the ligamentum transversum genu, and the anterior horn of medial meniscus (MM) without any obstacles (figures 7.3(c) and (d)). Finally, the cruciate ligament was cut, and the tibia and femur were split, the medial meniscus, the lateral meniscus (LM), the anterior horns of menisci, the posterior horns of menisci, and attachment point of cruciate ligament could be seen (figure 7.3(e)). These tissues were above the tibial plateau which was almost parallel to the x–y plane (i.e. the imaging plane). From these anatomical pictures, the dimensions of knee joint, cruciate ligament, lateral meniscus, and small ligament could be estimated to be 15, 3.8, 2.7, and 2 mm, respectively.

Since the imaging plane was almost identical to the tibial plateau plane, the resulting TAT image (figure 7.3(f)) should contain information primarily from the thin tibial plateau tissue with information from other tissues overlaid due to the relatively poor resolution along the z-axis. From figure 7.3(f), we can see that various joint tissues including ligamentum patellae, retinaculum patellae, fat pad, small ligament, ligamentum transversum genu, anterior horns of menisci, posterior horns of menisci, medial meniscus, lateral meniscus, posterior cruciate ligament, and anterior cruciate ligament can be detected by TAT, in comparison with the anatomical pictures. By estimating the full width at half maximum (FWHM) of the TAT image profiles shown in figures 7.3(k)–(n), the dimensions of the various recovered tissues were obtained to be 15.1, 3.9, 2.7, and 1.8 mm, respectively, for the whole knee joint, cruciate ligament, lateral meniscus, and small ligament. We noted that all these dimensions were in good agreement with the actual dimensions of these

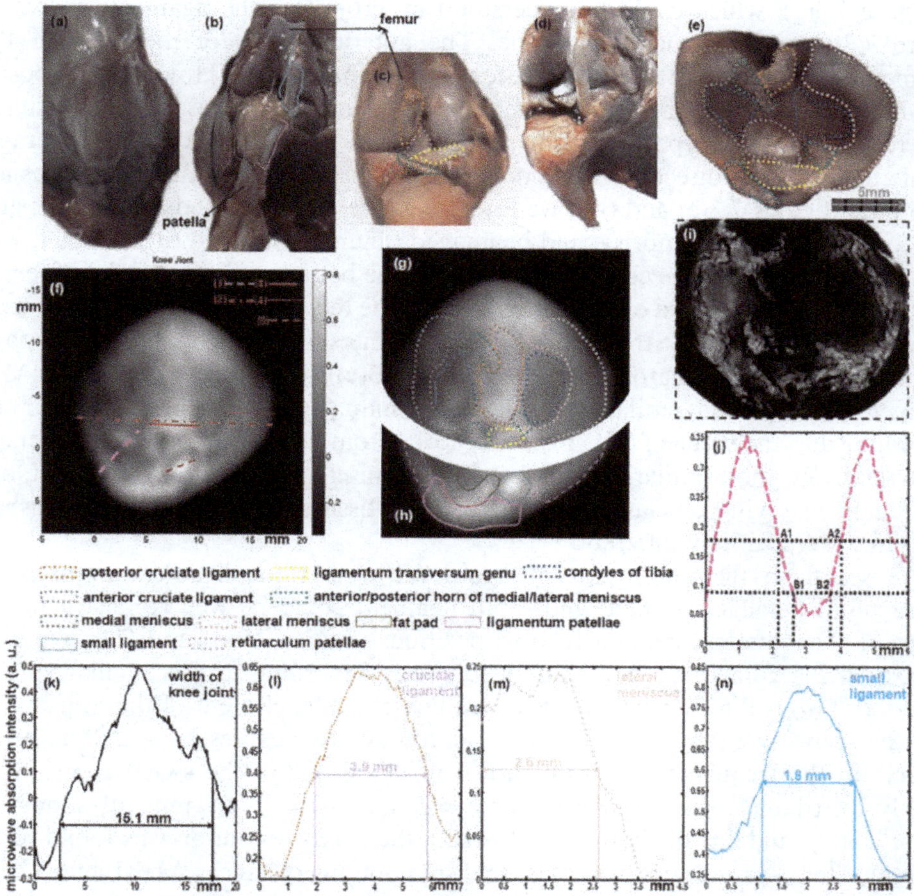

Figure 7.3. Comparison in TAT images and anatomical pictures of the left knee joint of a whole rabbit corpse. Anatomical pictures ((a)–(e)): the knee joint (without the skin) (a), and patella was stripped from femur (b), and fat pad was spun off ((c) and (d)), and several tissues on tibial plateau (e). TAT reconstruction images ((f)–(h)): a whole TAI reconstruction (f), and the image shown in figure 7.3(f) was divided in two parts ((g) and (h)). Structural similarity (SSIM) map (i) of the grayscale image of anatomical picture (e) without outlines, and reconstruction image without outlines (g). Recovered microwave absorption profiles ((j)–(n)): plotted along lines ((1)–(5)) from the image shown in figure 7.3(f), respectively. Reproduced from Chi *et al* (2016), © John Wiley & Sons.

tissues (the whole knee joint = 15 mm, cruciate ligament = 3.8 mm, lateral meniscus = 2.7 mm, and small ligament = 2 mm).

In order to have a better comparison with the anatomical pictures, the TAT image shown in figure 7.3(f) was separated into two parts, upper and lower parts (figures 7.3(g) and (h)). The menisci consisting of two semilunar fibrocartilaginous disks were reconstructed moderately from the upper part (figure 7.3(g)). In addition, the recovered MM appeared to be worse than the LM because MM was smaller in both size and thickness. This could be improved if a larger rotation angle was used for data collection. The anterior and posterior cruciate ligaments could be identified in figure 7.3(g), which could be understood by projecting the ligaments shown in figure 7.3(c) onto the imaging plane. The anterior horns of menisci and the ligamentum transversum genu were reconstructed moderately. However, the posterior horns of menisci image section were poorly recovered because very little signal was received from this portion of the tissues due to the limited scanning coverage. While there was no direct correspondence for the tissues highlighted by the dashed blue lines (figures 7.3(e) and (g)), we found that the condylus medialis femoris and the condylus lateralis femoris could be imaged (figures 7.3(c) and (d)). Thus, it was reasonable to say that the condyles of femur or the boundaries of condyles of femur were most likely projected onto the inner side of the recovered menisci. We also used a structural similarity (SSIM) index to measure the similarity between TAT image (figure 7.3(g)) and the anatomical image (figure 7.3(e)). The highest value of SSIM is 1 which shows perfect similarity. In the SSIM map (figure 7.3(i)), the brighter the color indicates the value of SSIM is closer to 1. From figure 7.3(i), we see that there were relatively good similarities involving the menisci and the horns of menisci, but the region involving cruciate ligaments and the tissues highlighted by the dashed blue lines were entirely different.

We see from the lower part of figure 7.3(h) that the ligamentum patellae, retinaculum patellae, fat pad, and small ligament could be well reconstructed in terms of their dimensions and relative positions (figures 7.3(a) and (b)). We also calculated the z-axis and x–y plane resolution. According to the angular spread formula $\sin(\theta) = 0.61\ \lambda/r$, where r is the radius of active element of the transducer, and the scanning radius R, the z-axis resolution can be expressed as $2R^*\tan(\theta)$ in theory. In the frequency spectrum shown in figure 7.2(d), the signal spectrum is mainly distributed under 2 MHz. For $r = 3$ mm, $R = 114.5$ mm (as shown in figure 7.3(e)), and $\lambda = 0.75$ mm ($f = 2$ MHz), the z-axis resolution was found to be 3.5 mm. The x–y resolution was measured by summing distances A1-B1 and A2-B2 (A1 and A2: points at half maximum, and B1 and B2: points at quarter maximum) from the reconstruction profile given in figure 7.3(j). The profile here in figure 7.3(j) was obtained along line (1) crossing through retinaculum patellae and medial meniscus, as shown in figure 7.3(f). Based on this criterion, the x–y resolution was calculated to be 0.75 mm.

The spatial resolution was determined by the system as well as the specific imaging object of interest (Nie *et al* 2008). Owing to the complexity of joint tissues and large differences in their acoustic impedances, the effect caused by acoustic reflections cannot be ignored. For example, some of the thermoacoustic signals produced by joint soft tissues reached the detector after being reflected from bones instead of reaching the detector directly, which could change the TA signal in amplitude and phase. The distorted signals could then cause both blurring and reduced contrast in the resulting TA image. Also, the higher frequency components attenuated faster compared with the lower frequency ones, which could adversely affect the imaging resolution.

An attempt was also made to estimate the microwave absorption coefficients of joint tissues for the recovered TAT images using the following equation:

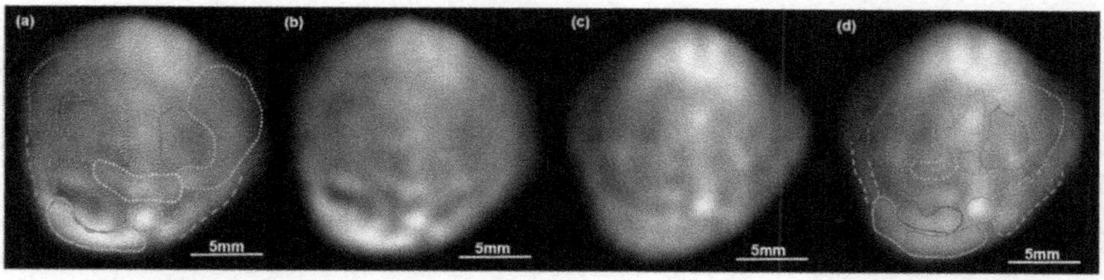

Figure 7.4. *In vivo* reconstruction images of rabbit knee joint in two different postures: one posture ((a) and (b)) and the other posture ((c) and (d)). The general outlines of the knee joint tissues for (b) and (c) are drawn in (a) and (d), respectively. Outline of different colors represents different tissues, similar to figure 7.3. Reproduced from Chi *et al* (2016), © John Wiley & Sons.

$$\alpha = \omega\sqrt{\frac{\mu\varepsilon}{2}\left[\sqrt{1+\left(\frac{\sigma}{\omega\mu}\right)^2}-1\right]} \tag{7.1}$$

where ω is the angular frequency of microwave, μ is the permeability, ε is the dielectric constant, and σ is the conductivity. In our imaging system, the magnetic properties could be ignored and the microwave absorption coefficients were mainly determined by the dielectric properties (Wang *et al* 2012). We first approximately calculated the theoretical values of α_{ligament} and α_{meniscus}, and then estimated these two parameters using the recovered TAT images. The relative permittivity and the conductivity are 42.13 and 2.17 S m^{-1}, and 37.61 and 2.21 S m^{-1}, respectively, for tendon and cartilage from *ex vivo* animal or human tissues. As ligaments and tendons have almost the same composition (Paessler and Mastrokalos 2003), the conductivity of the ligament was assumed to be similar to that of the tendon in this study. Thus, the ratio between the absorption coefficients of ligament and meniscus could be calculated as $\alpha_{\text{ligament}}/\alpha_{\text{meniscus}} = 0.93$. This ratio could also be estimated from the reconstructed TAT images. While TAT directly detects microwave energy absorption distribution (i.e. the product of absorption coefficient and radiated energy), here we could assume that TAT imaged the tissue absorption coefficients equivalently as the distance between small ligament and lateral meniscus was so close that the microwave energy was almost equal in these two regions (Fu *et al* 2014, Ding *et al* 2015). From figures 7.3(m) and (n), we noted that the average values for ligament and meniscus were $TA_{\text{ligament}} = 0.57$ and $TA_{\text{meniscus}} = 0.13$, respectively. Considering a *z*-axis resolution of 3.5 mm, $\alpha'_{\text{ligament}} \approx TA_{\text{ligament}}/3.5 = 0.16$ mm. As the cross section of meniscus is triangular, and its outer thickness was about 1 mm, $\alpha'_{\text{meniscus}} \approx TA_{\text{meniscus}}/1 = 0.13$/mm. Thus, we had $\alpha'_{\text{ligament}} \approx/\alpha'_{\text{meniscus}}$ meniscus = 1.23, which was in agreement with the theoretical value. Tissue absorption coefficient may be related to tissue functional information (Nie *et al* 2008), which suggests that TAT has the potential to diagnose joint diseases at an early stage.

Figures 7.4(b) and (c) show the TAT images obtained when the left knee joint of one rabbit was in two different postures. This needed to be examined as the anesthetized knee joint could still move while it was kept in a genuflex position for data collection. We immediately noted the differences in image quality from figures 7.4(b) and (c). In general, the image shown in figure 7.4(b) presents better recovery of joint tissues; however, the differences are not considerable as the major joint tissues could also be identified (figure 7.4(a) and (d)).

Figures 7.5(a) and (d) show the TAT images obtained from two rabbits, one that was dead just before the TAT imaging, and the other that was gaining consciousness from the anesthetization during the imaging. Clearly, figures 7.5(a) and (b) show better image quality, while motion effect-associated noise blurred the image (figure 7.5(d)). In both cases, the major joint tissues could be identified, see figures 7.5(b) and (c).

Figure 7.6 presents the TAI images obtained when the scanning was performed at 7 different positions along the z-axis (an x–y–z coordinate system is shown in figure 7.6(h)). Given the relatively poor resolution along the z-axis, the differences among these images are still notable although not large. For example, the images shown in figures 7.6(a) and (g) are significantly different as they clearly accounted for contributions from different joint tissues. The use of a line-focused transducer would certainly improve the resolution along the z-axis, thus the image quality at different scanning positions along this direction.

7.1.2 Healthy human finger joints

7.1.2.1 Participants

Reprinted, with permission from IEEE, from Chi *et al* (2019).

All the participating volunteers provided written informed consent. Eight healthy middle and index fingers from five volunteers were imaged *in vivo* by our TAT imaging system. Axial T1-weighted MR imaging (3.0T) was used to validate the TAT findings. Comparative analyses between TAT and MRI images were performed in two dimensions for all the fingers imaged. Three-dimensional (3D) images and animations were also obtained for some of the fingers thermoacoustically scanned.

These healthy volunteers (mean age = 27 years; range = 25–31 years) had no history of arthritic conditions or clinical evidence of peripheral joint involvement, and were coded as: HM1, HM2, and HM3 for 3 healthy males; HF1 and HF2 for 2 healthy females. A total of eight healthy fingers (three right middle fingers from HM1, HM2, and HF1, two right index fingers from HM3 and HF1, two left middle

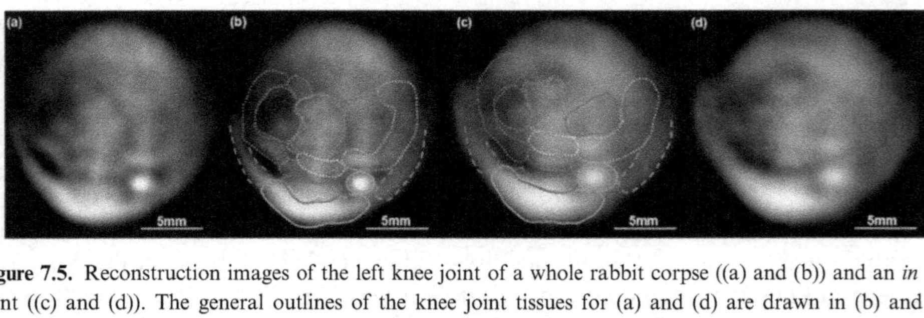

Figure 7.5. Reconstruction images of the left knee joint of a whole rabbit corpse ((a) and (b)) and an *in vivo* joint ((c) and (d)). The general outlines of the knee joint tissues for (a) and (d) are drawn in (b) and (c), respectively. Outlines of different colors represent different tissues, similar to figure 7.3. Reproduced from Chi *et al* (2016), © John Wiley & Sons.

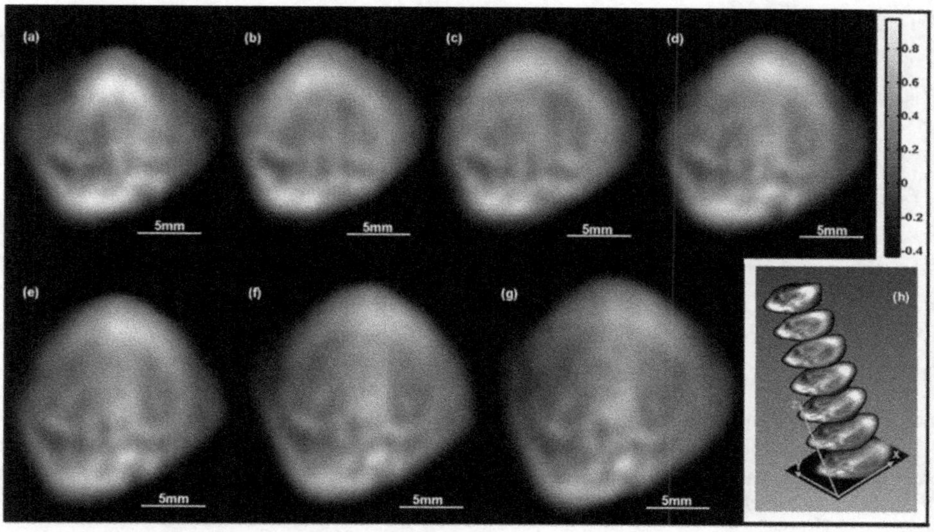

Figure 7.6. TAI images at different scanning positions along the *z*-axis. The interval between two adjacent scans was 2 mm. Reproduced from Chi *et al* (2016), © John Wiley & Sons.

fingers from HF1 and HF2, and one left index finger from HF1) were imaged by TAT. We considered the following two aspects to ensure the reproducibility: different fingers for the same subject, and similar fingers for different subjects. Four subjects (HM1, HM2, HM3, and HF1) were examined with MRI as well (HF2 was not available for MR scan at the time).

7.1.2.2 TAT system

The TAT system used for joint imaging includes microwave pulse generation and delivery, arrangement for hand and finger placement, thermoacoustic signal receiving, and image reconstruction, as shown in figure 7.7, where an x–y–z coordinate system is also indicated. A custom-designed microwave generator coupled with a waveguide-feed pyramidal horn antenna (aperture size: 114×144 mm^2) was used to provide a pulsed microwave (frequency: 3.0 GHz, bandwidth: 50 MHz, peak power: 70 kW, and pulse duration: 750 ns), which shone onto the object from the above. The microwave power density at the object surface was measured to be less than the safety standard (100 W m^{-2} at 3 GHz). In this study, no skin damage, side effects, or any adverse events resulted from the TAT imaging procedures.

The hand and fingers of the volunteer were placed in a holder consisting of two parts (upper part: holder 1, and lower part: holder 2, as shown in figure 7.7(a)) to avoid potential motion artifacts in TAT imaging. The tip of the middle finger being imaged was fixed at holder 1 (connected with the antenna), while other fingers were put in holder 2 located at the bottom of the tank (figures 7.7(b) and (c)). When an index finger was being imaged, holder 3 was used to replace holder 2 (figures 7.7(d) and (e)). Due to individual differences in dimensions of the fingers, different holders were used for each subject, and fine tuning of the finger positioning was required to

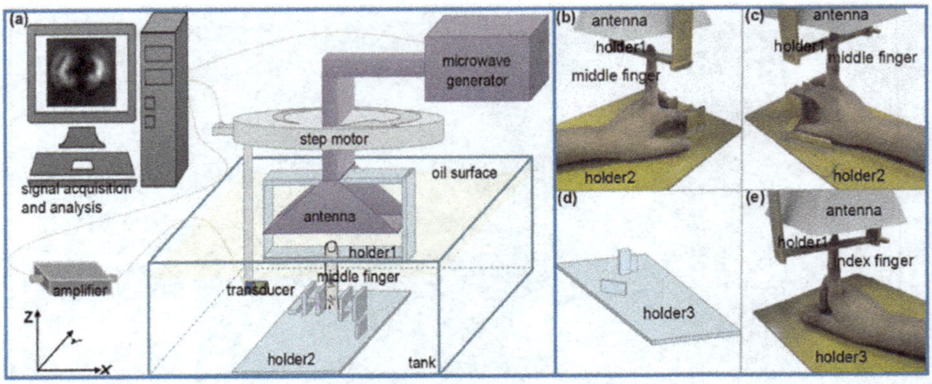

Figure 7.7. TAT imaging system and hand/fingers positioning. (a) Schematic of the TAT system. (b) and (c): photograph showing the left and right middle finger being imaged, respectively. (d) and (e): holder 3 and photograph showing the right index finger being imaged. © 2019 IEEE. Reprinted, with permission, from Chi *et al* (2019).

ensure a good alignment of the finger being imaged with the propagation direction of the microwave (i.e. along the *z*-axis).

During the TAT imaging, the hand and the finger being imaged (except for the tip), and most of the arm were immersed in a tank filled with mineral oil, which served as a coupling medium for high efficiency transmission of the microwave and acoustic signals. The ultrasonic signals produced by the tissue absorption of microwave energy were detected by a 5 MHz cylindrically focused ultrasound transducer (V326, Olympus; active-element diameter: 10 mm; focal length: 53 mm). To realize 2D cross sectional imaging of the finger, the transducer rotated around the finger horizontally in the *x*–*y* plane with a radius of 7 mm. To cover a 360° receiving angle, 180 transducer positions with a constant interval of 2° were used. After being amplified by a homemade amplifier (voltage gain: 58.7 dB; −3 dB bandwidth: 570 kHz–2 MHz), the detected acoustic signal was sampled and averaged 50 times to achieve a good SNR by data acquisition card (PCI4732, Vidts Dynamic). Labview programming was used to control the entire examination procedure. Finally, the thermoacoustic signals acquired at different transducer positions were used to form the tissue dielectric property distribution using a delay-and-sum algorithm. To achieve 3D imaging of the finger, multiple 2D cross-sectional images were acquired along the *z*-axis with an interval of 2 mm. Based on the parameters of the transducer used, the theoretical axial resolution of our TAT system was 1.6 mm.

The repetition frequency of microwave pulse was set to be 100 Hz and the time needed for cross-sectional scanning of a single finger was about 90 s (excluding a time of ~30 s for preparation/finger positioning). To eliminate possible artifacts due to motions and fatigue as a result of a long signal acquisition, a time of up to 10 min resting was used between two adjacent scans. Cross-sectional scanning at each transducer position was repeated three times to guarantee the repeatability. Therefore, it took more than 10 hours to scan a whole finger. In our TAT

Table 7.1. The actual joints and number of cross sectional TAT scanning performed for each subject. © 2019 IEEE. Reprinted, with permission, from Chi *et al* (2019).

Subject	HM1	HM2	HM3	HF1	HF1	HF1	HF1	HF2
Finger	RM	RM	RI	RM	RI	LM	LI	LM
PP	Partial	Partial	Partial	Partial	Partial	Partial	Partial	Partial
PIP	Whole	Whole	Whole	Whole	Whole	Whole	Whole	Whole
MP	Partial	Partial	Whole	Whole	Whole	Whole	Whole	Partial
DIP	—	—	Partial	Partial	Partial	Partial	Partial	—
Number of scans	16	17	17	25	21	23	19	16

HM1–HM3 and HF1–HF2 stand for the three male and two female volunteers, respectively; RM = right middle finger, RI = right index finger, LM = left middle finger, and LI = left index finger; PP = proximal phalanx, DIP = distal interphalangeal joint, MP = middle phalanx, and PIP = proximal interphalangeal joint.

experiments, the actual number of joints imaged and/or cross-sectional scanning used was different for different volunteers, as detailed in table 7.1.

7.1.2.3 Magnetic resonance imaging

To validate the anatomic structures visualized in axial TAT cross-sectional images, axial T1-weighed spin-echo sequence was performed (Erickson *et al* 1989, Gupta *et al* 2015). The specific parameters used for MR scans were as follows: repetition time ms/echo time ms, 500/10; FOV, 120 mm; thickness mm /spacing mm, 3.5/0.5; matrix, 256 × 256; number of sections, 25; and Nex, 2. MRI examination of the fingers was performed on a 3.0-T scanner (GE Discovery MRI 750) by using a single-channel knee-and-foot coil. During the exam, the subject was placed in a prone position, with the hands fixed over the head with the help of several cushions, while the whole index and middle fingers were located simultaneously in the field of view (FoV). MRI scanning of each hand required ~5 min.

7.1.2.4 Image analyses

Based on the MR images, we drew and distinguished the different dashed lines along the alternate boundary between light and dark regions in TAT images. Detailed structural comparative analyses between the TAT and the corresponding MRI images involving both the PP and PIP joints were performed. According to the TAT images of the PP, the *x*–*y* plane resolution was evaluated. To demonstrate the reproducibility, TAT images about articular surfaces of several PIPs from different volunteers were presented and analyzed. According to the TAT images of the PIP, the contrast of different finger structures was estimated.

For the MP and DIP joints, comparative analyses and reproducibility validation were also performed. The 2D axial TAT images of an entire finger containing partial DIP, whole MP, whole PIP and partial PP, were presented. 3D reconstruction and animation of this entire finger were acquired with software Amira (version 5.3.3, TGS Template Graphics Software) and Photoshop (Adobe Photoshop c.c. 2015), respectively.

7.1.2.5 *Results*

7.1.2.5.1 Proximal interphalangeal joint and proximal phalanx

The 2D TAT and MR images of the whole PIP and partial PP of the middle finger for HM1 are presented side-by-side in figure 7.8. The interval between two adjacent TAT scans and MR scans was 2 and 4 mm, respectively. As shown in figure 7.8(a),

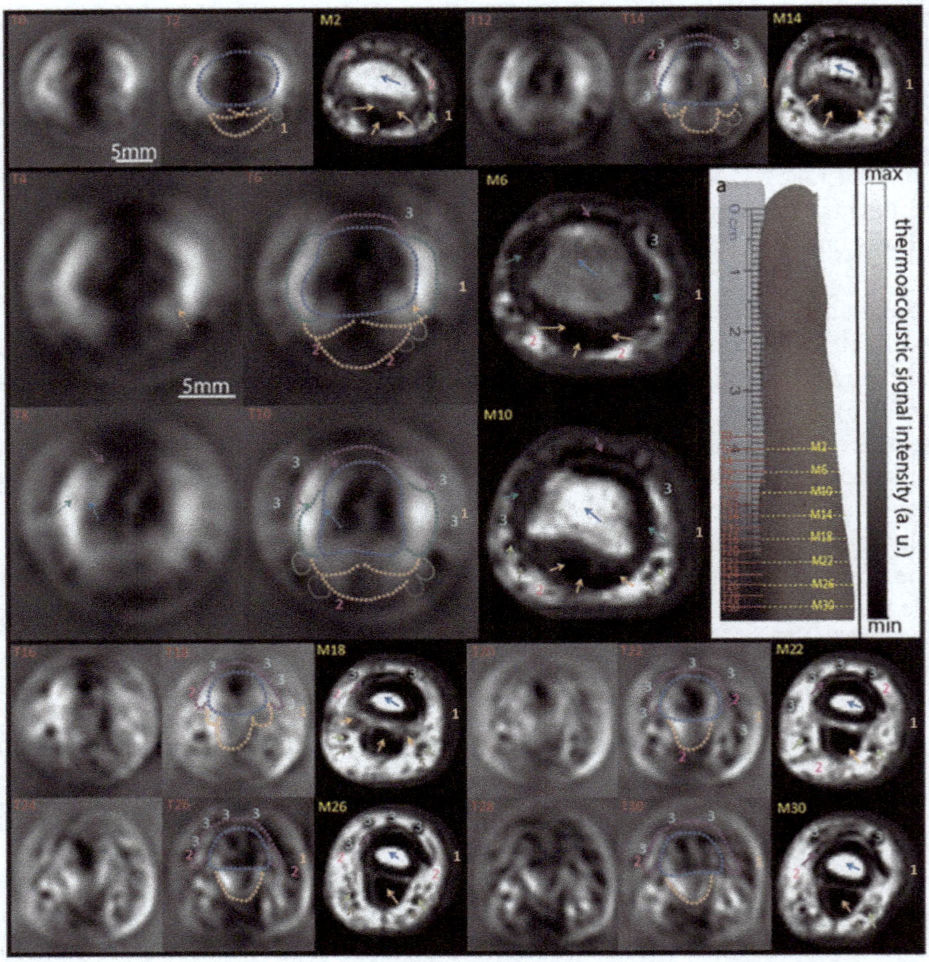

Figure 7.8. Comparison of TAT and MR images of the middle finger for a representative subject (HM1). 16 TAT images (T0–T30): the spatial interval between two adjacent slices was 2 mm. Eight MR images (M2–M30): the spatial interval between two adjacent slices was 4 mm. (a) Photograph of the finger being imaged and the measure showing the imaging cross-sectional positions for both TAT and MRI. Colored numbers and marks in some of the above images: 1-skin, 2-subcutaneous fat, 3-blood vessel, ⇢ proper palmar digital artery, ⇢ proper palmar digital nerve, ⇢ flexor tendon, ⇢ extensor tendon, ⇢ collateral ligament, ⇢ bone, ⇢ space between bone and collateral ligament, ⇢ space between collateral ligament and extensor tendon, ⇢ space between extensor tendon and bone, ⇢ space between flexor tendon and bone. © 2019 IEEE. Reprinted, with permission, from Chi *et al* (2019).

the 16 TAT images were numbered in sequence as T0, T2, T4,… and T30, while the eight MR images were numbered in sequence as M2, M6,… and M30.

In TAT images, the skin was identified as indicated by number 1. Clinging to the skin were some dark and bright regions as noted by numbers 2 and 3, which were subcutaneous fat and blood vessels, respectively. These three types of tissues were marked by the same numbers in the corresponding MR images, where we see that in contrast, the subcutaneous fat and blood vessels showed bright and dark in MR signal. The proper palmar digital artery, proper palmar digital nerve, flexor tendon, extensor tendon, collateral ligament and bone were all distinguishable and noted by dotted outlines of different colors in several of the TAT images. These tissues were marked by arrows of the corresponding colors in the MR images.

In figure 7.8(T0)–(T22), the flexor tendon (FT) (figure 7.8(T20)–(T22)) outlined by the orange dotted lines was gradually distinguished into flexor digitorum profundus tendon (FDPT) (the central orange dotted lines) and flexor digitorum superficialis tendon (FDST) (the bilateral orange dotted lines), respectively (figure 7.8(T0)–(T18)). Along the outward direction of the finger, the FDST tissues tended to be separated first and then merged together. Volar plate between the FDST and bone at the joint could not be clearly distinguished from the FDST. Retinaculum located near the green dotted line was not differentiated from the striking contributor-collateral ligament (outlined by the green dotted line). Thus, both volar plate and retinaculum were not marked in the images shown in figure 7.8.

The articular surface (outlined by the blue dotted line) was accurately localized in the TAT images (figure 7.8(T4)–(T10)), which matched well with the position of PIP joint in the photograph of the finger shown in figure 7.8(a). The articular surface is the bone surface that forms the joint, while the articular surface is covered by articular cartilage. The area indicated by the blue dotted lines included both the cancellous bone and cartilage, while the signal from the cartilage was be considered to be stronger than the bone because the cartilage had higher dielectric properties (Gabriel *et al* 1996a, 1996b). The spaces among the bone, collateral ligament and tendon were clearly marked by the dotted arrows in figure 7.8(T4)–(T10). These spaces were considered as the location of synovium because all the intra-articular ligaments, bones, and tendons should be covered by the synovium.

The bone was identified by the areas indicated by the numbers 4 and 5 in TAT image (figures 7.9(a)–(c)), in comparison with the MR image (figures 7.9(a-1)–(b-1)). These areas overlap partially with the cortical bone and marrow cavity. While we believe these areas were bone structures, the determination of the specific types of bones warrants further studies. Compared to the MR image shown in figure 7.9(a-1)–(b-1), the tissues enclosed by the black lines in figures 7.9(a)–(c) indicated the proper palmar digital artery and proper palmar digital nerve.

The x–y resolution was measured by summing the distances A1-B1 and A2-B2 (A1 and A2: points at the half maximum; B1 and B2: points at the quarter maximum) from the TAT profiles given in figures 7.9(d)–(g) and taking the average of the four values. The profiles here in figures 7.9(d)–(g) were obtained along four lines (I), (II), (III), and (IV) as shown in figures 7.9(a)–(c), respectively. The x–y resolution was calculated to be 0.37 mm.

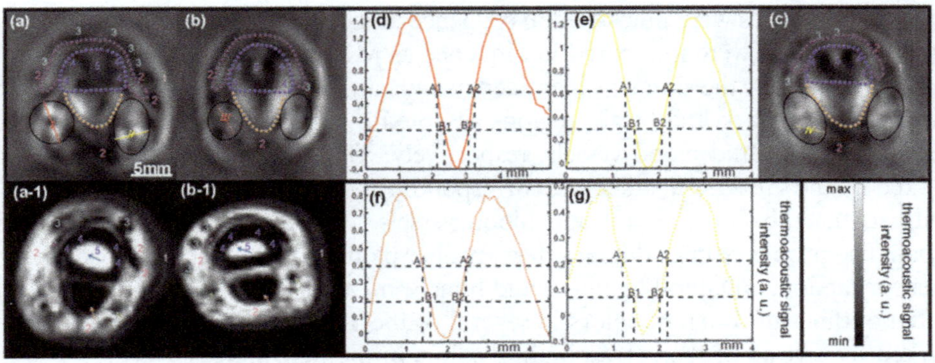

Figure 7.9. Detailed analysis of the cross section shown in figure 7.8(T28) and the resolution calculation. TAT images ((a), (b), and (c)) and MR images ((a-1) and (b-1)) for 3 volunteers: HM1((a) and (a-1)), HF1 ((b) and (b-1)) and HF2 (c). Recovered thermoacoustic signal intensity profiles ((d)-(g)): plotted along lines ((I)-(IV)) from the images shown in figures 7.9(a)–(c), respectively. © 2019 IEEE. Reprinted, with permission, from Chi *et al* (2019).

The PIP articular surfaces of the middle finger for four volunteers were accurately imaged and are presented in figure 7.10. Intra-articular tissues containing extensor tendon, collateral ligament, flexor tendon and bone are well distinguished by the dotted outlines of different colors. The spaces enclosing synovium are also marked by the dotted arrows.

Partial information inside each articular surface outlined by the blue dotted lines were missing, due to the loss of low frequency signal given the limited frequency response of the transducers used in TAT imaging (Xi and Jiang 2016). Differences existed among different articular surfaces, resulted by the acoustic reflections from the bone. The reflected signals would be weakened to different extent and would most affect deeply located tissues (Biswas *et al* 2015, Deng and Li 2016).

The imaging contrast was estimated. TAT directly detects thermoacoustic signal intensity distribution (i.e. the product of absorption coefficient and radiated energy) (Fu *et al* 2014, Ding *et al* 2015). We computed pixel mean values of several colored rectangle boxes shown in figure 7.11(a). These values were plotted in figure 7.11(b) to show the thermoacoustic signal intensity of the corresponding structures. The theoretical microwave absorption coefficients of tissues (figure 7.11(c)) were obtained by using equation (7.1). The relative permittivity and the conductivity of tissues were obtained through the literature from *ex vivo* animal or human tissues (Gabriel *et al* 1996a, 1996b).

The general trend of thermoacoustic signal intensity (figure 7.11(b)) for most tissue types was consistent with that of theoretical absorption coefficients (figure 7.11(c)) excepted for the cartilage. Three main reasons were taken into account. Cartilage thickness along the z-axis was thin, which may be less than the axial resolution centered on the imaging plane. Partial information involving cartilage and bone was missing due to the limited frequency response of the transducers (see the detailed analysis for figure 7.10). Experimental results involved contrast deteriorations because of inhomogeneous radiated energy and acoustic reflections due to inhomogeneous acoustic media.

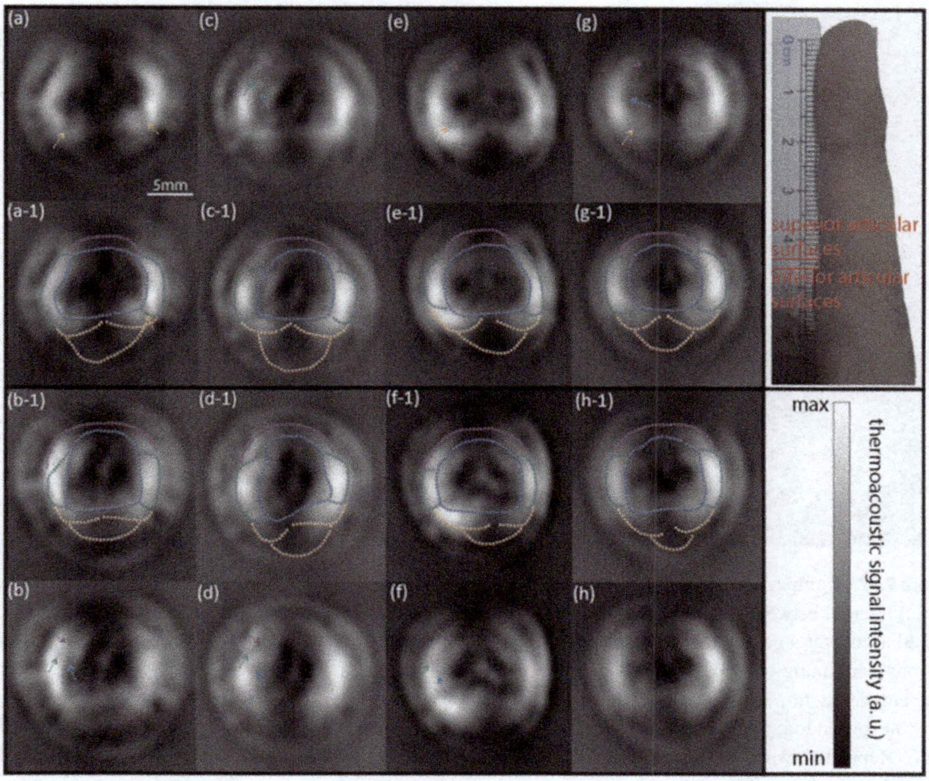

Figure 7.10. TAT images of PIP articular surfaces of the middle finger for four volunteers. Right middle finger: HM1 ((a), (a-1), (b), and (b-1)), and HM2 ((c), (c-1), (d), and (d-1)). Left middle finger: HF1 ((e), (e-1), (f), and (f-1)), and HF2 ((g), (g-1), (h), and (h-1)). Superior articular surfaces ((a), (a-1), (c), (c-1),(e), (e-1),(g), and (g-1)). Inferior articular surfaces ((b), (b-1), (d), (d-1),(f), (f-1),(h), and (h-1)). The general outlines of the PIP joint tissues for (a)–(h) are drawn in (a-1)–(h-1). The spaces among the bone, collateral ligament and tendon are marked in (a)–(h). Outlines of different colors represent different tissues, similar to that in figure 7.8. © 2019 IEEE. Reprinted, with permission, from Chi *et al* (2019).

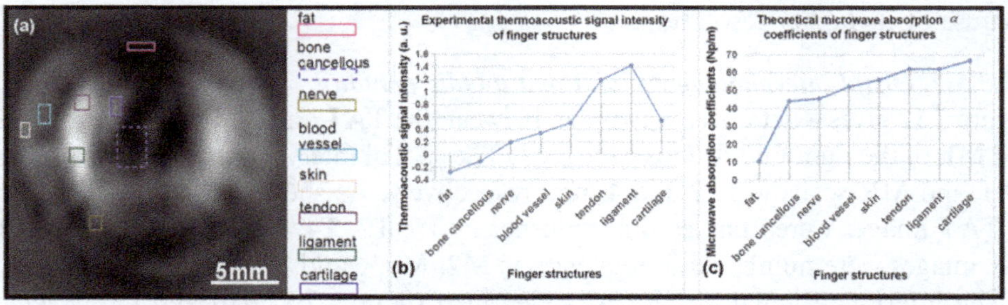

Figure 7.11. The contrast estimations of different finger structures shown in figure 7.10(b). Pixel mean values of several colored rectangle boxes shown in figure 7.11(a) were computed as the experimental thermoacoustic signal intensity for the finger structures shown in figure 7.11(b). Theoretical microwave absorption coefficients of different finger structures are presented in figure 7.11(c). © 2019 IEEE. Reprinted, with permission, from Chi *et al* (2019).

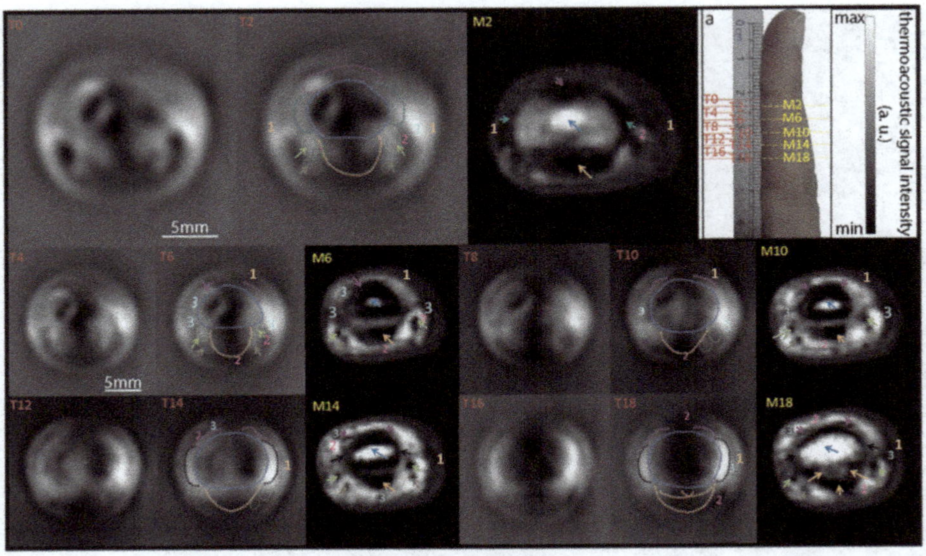

Figure 7.12. Comparison in TAT and MR images of the middle finger for HF1. TAT images ((T0)–(T18)): the spatial interval between two adjacent slices was 2 mm. MR images ((M2)–(M18)): the spatial interval between two adjacent was 4 mm. (a) Photograph of the finger being imaged and the measure showing the imaging cross sections containing the DIP and MP. Colored numbers and marks in some of the above images: 1-skin, 2-subcutaneous fat, 3-blood vessel, → proper palmar digital artery, → proper palmar digital nerve, → flexor tendon, → extensor tendon, → collateral ligament, → bone, → retinaculum. © 2019 IEEE. Reprinted, with permission, from Chi *et al* (2019).

When a disease occurs, accompanied by some changes in composition, the dielectric properties of the tissue will also change. In osteoporosis, the lost bone mass is replaced by fat (low dielectric properties) and bone marrow (high dielectric properties) (Zhou *et al* 2010). Overall, injured bones show higher dielectric properties than normal ones in microwave imaging (MI) (Golnabi *et al* 2011). For MI of damaged *ex vivo* ligaments, tendons or cartilage, the differential maps can locate the lesions with low dielectric properties (Salvador *et al* 2009a, 2009b). Similarly, based on the differences in tissue dielectric properties, TAT may perform better than MI because of its higher resolution.

7.1.2.5.2 Distal interphalangeal joint and middle phalanx

Figure 7.12 gives a detailed comparison between the TAT and MR images of the DIP and MP of the right middle finger for HF1. The spatial intervals between two adjacent TAT and MR scans were 2 and 4 mm, respectively. As shown in figure 7.12(a), the 10 TAT images were numbered in sequence as T0, T2, T4,…and T18, while the five MR images were numbered in sequence as M2, M6,…and M18.

The inferior articular surface was identified (figures 7.12(T0) and (T2)), which matched well with the position of DIP joint (figure 7.12(a)). Various tissues delineated are marked in figure 7.12. Compared to the PIP, the spaces among the bone, collateral ligament and tendon were not clearly imaged in part due to the smaller size of DIP. However, the boundaries of these spaces could still be detected, which helped locate the synovium.

The DIP inferior articular surfaces for five different fingers from two volunteers were accurately delineated (figure 7.13). Intra-articular tissues containing extensor tendon, collateral ligament, flexor tendon and bone were all distinguishable (see the dotted outlines of different colors in figure 7.13).

7.1.2.5.3 Whole finger

Twelve axial TAT slices along the whole left middle finger for HF1 are presented in figure 7.14. These slices show the structural differences/changes along the axial direction of the finger, while they also demonstrate consistency compared to some of the images shown in figures 7.8 and 7.12 on similar joints.

To better display the stereoscopic effect of the extension and transformation of the inner part of the finger along the axis, 3D image reconstruction was performed and the 3D rendering is given in figure 7.15. The 3D rendering shows that the overall structure was well recovered compared to the photograph of the finger, and in figure 7.15(b1) the proper palmar digital artery and proper palmar digital nerve were clearly identified. We also see that the artery and nerve travel to the fingertip from the root along both sides of the finger. The flexor tendon was imaged and marked in figures 7.15(a) and (b1).

7.1.2.6 Discussion

TAT can recover various joint tissues (both soft and hard tissues). Tendons and ligaments, often involved in traumatic joint injuries, are well visualized in TAT images (figure 7.8) (Wieschhoff *et al* 2016). Synovium is located at the space between ligament/tendon and bone/cartilage at the articular cavity (figure 7.10). Synovitis is a key characteristic of any arthritic diseases (Balakrishnan *et al* 2014). It should be noted that the synovium itself is not detected here because healthy synovium is very thin (less than 100 μm) (Van Es *et al* 2015). The inflamed synovium edema and

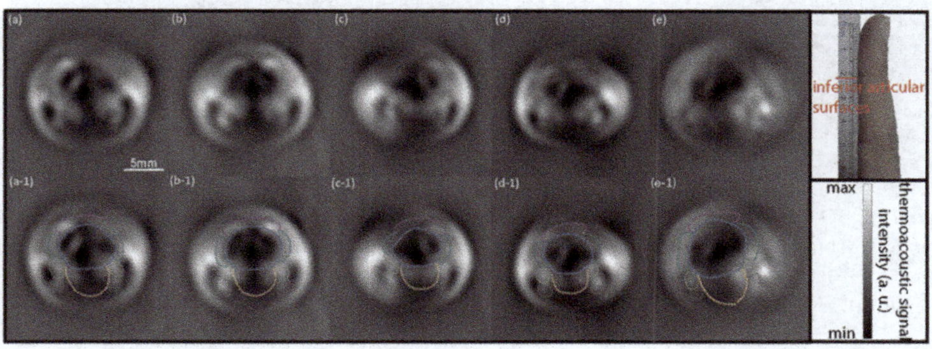

Figure 7.13. TAT images of DIP inferior articular surfaces for five different fingers from two volunteers. Middle fingers from HF1: right ((a) and (a1)), and left ((b) and (b1)). Index fingers from HF1: left ((c) and (c1)), and right ((d) and (d1)). Index fingers from HM3 ((e) and (e1)). (a1)-(d1) give the outlines of the DIP joint tissues identified in (a)-(d). Outlines of different colors represent different tissues, similar to figure 7.12. © 2019 IEEE. Reprinted, with permission, from Chi *et al* (2019).

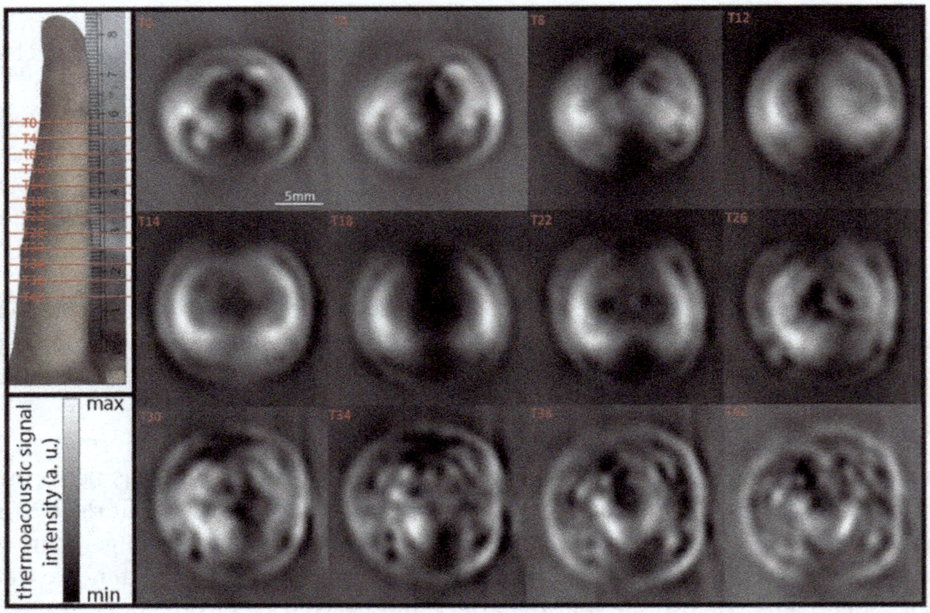

Figure 7.14. TAT images at different scanning positions along the axis of the left middle finger for HF1. The spatial interval between two adjacent scans was 4 mm. © 2019 IEEE. Reprinted, with permission, from Chi *et al* (2019).

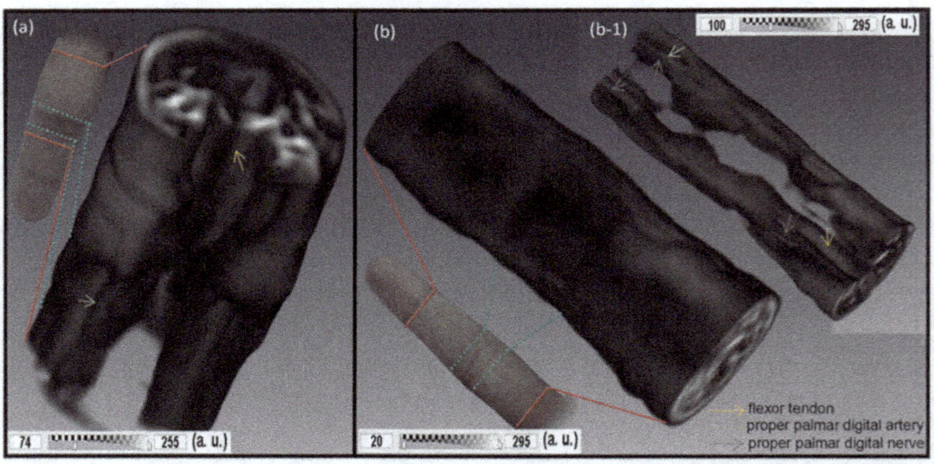

Figure 7.15. 3D image reconstruction. Half finger containing the whole PIP and partial PP of the right middle finger for HM1 (a); whole finger containing partial DIP, whole MP, whole PIP and partial PP of the left middle finger for HF1 ((b) and (b1)). Varying degrees of threshold values used in the reconstruction: mild (b); moderate (a); severe (b1). © 2019 IEEE. Reprinted, with permission, from Chi *et al* (2019).

thickening accompanied by elevated inflammatory ions and water content may have increased conductivity. Meanwhile, a thicker synovium has a stronger signal at a lower frequency (Van Es *et al* 2015).

In addition to the soft tissues, TAT can recover the structures related to the bone. The areas overlapped partially with cortical bone and marrow cavity are well located (figure 7.9). The articular surface covered by cartilage can be imaged by TAT as well (figures 7.10 and 7.13). Cartilage is first damaged in joint diseases such as osteoarthritis (Hart and Spector 2000). Previous studies have shown that abnormal bone and cartilage can generate changes in dielectric properties (Salvador *et al* 2009a, 2009b, Golnabi *et al* 2011, Zhou *et al* 2010). Therefore, determination of specific types of bone and visualization of bone marrow edema will be another focus of our future research.

For TAT images of similar cross sections of different sexes, there is little difference in terms of the reconstructed structures (figures 7.10 and 7.13). Probably a major difference is that the images for a male finger joint (figure 7.10(a)–(d) and figure 7.13(e)) show larger sizes and more distinct layers than that of a female finger joint (figures 7.10(e)–(h) and figures 7.13(a)–(d)) in similar cross sections.

Differences are noted between the TAT and MRI images shown in figures 7.8, 7.9 and 7.12, and are explained as follows. First, the contrast mechanisms are different for TAT and MRI: TAT contrast is based on tissue microwave absorption, while MRI contrast is based on tissue T1 relaxation. Second, the TAT and MRI slices given might not be from the exact same cross-section, where the elevation resolution was different for the two modalities. Finally, the soft tissues involving the skin, subcutaneous fat and blood vessel were squeezed by cushions to avoid motion artifacts during the MR scans, while no compression was needed during the TAT scans.

Although the TAT images shown here have lower resolution relative to MRI, they allow us to effectively visualize the anatomic structures of the *in vivo* human finger joints. MRI needs to use contrast agent to assess the presence and amount of active synovitis (Mohajerani *et al* 2014, Plotkin *et al* 2016). TAT can easily locate the healthy thin synovium (figures 7.10 and 7.13) without the use of any contrast agent. Moreover, TAT imaging is relatively inexpensive and can be made quantitative in terms of tissue conductivity (Huang *et al* 2012, Yao *et al* 2010). We will apply TAT to detect and long-term monitor the changes in synovitic activity in a future study.

Compared with x-ray and CT which can image bone perfectly, non-ionizing TAT can preferably reconstruct soft tissue based on the contrast of tissue dielectric property. In addition, soft tissue is often easily damaged at an earlier stage for joint diseases. Compared with US, TAT is better for bone imaging because the ultrasound signal only needs to pass the bone once for TAT.

7.1.3 Diseased human finger joints

Here we present a pilot clinical study on TAT of rheumatoid arthritis in the finger joints using the imager shown in figure 7.7. Figure 7.16 gives the TAT images of the PIP joint of the left middle finger for a healthy volunteer (H#1), while figures 7.17 and 7.18 show the TAT images of the PIP joint of the left middle finger for patients #1 and #2 (R#1 and R#2). This healthy volunteer (age = 46 years) had no history of arthritic conditions or clinical evidence of peripheral joint involvement. As shown in

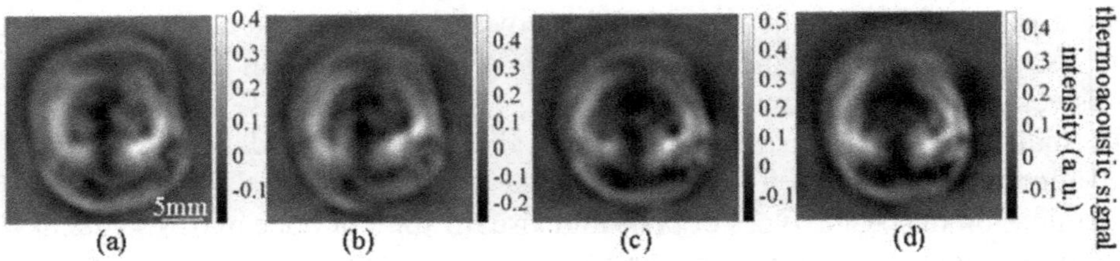

Figure 7.16. TAT images of the PIP joint of the left middle finger for H#1. (a)–(d) are cross-sectional images of the joint with a spatial interval of 2mm between two adjacent slices.

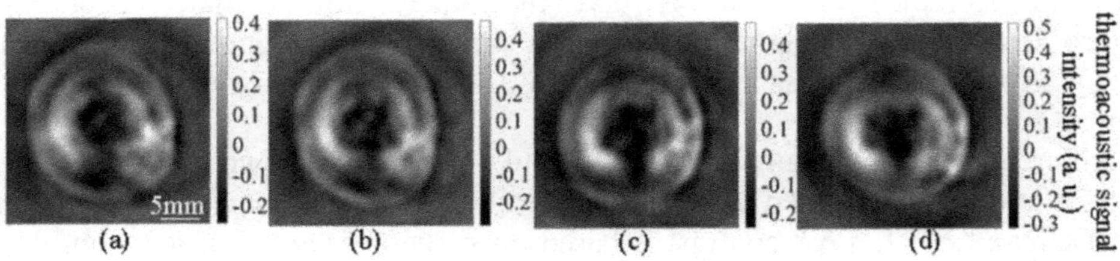

Figure 7.17. TAT images of the PIP joint of the left middle finger for R#1. (a)–(d) are cross-sectional images of the joint with a spatial interval of 2mm between two adjacent slices.

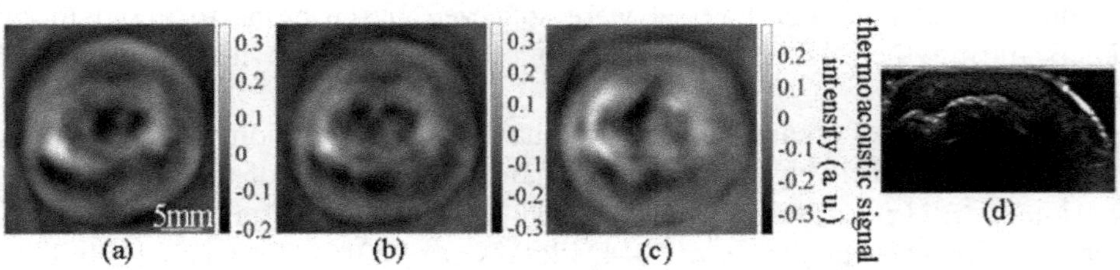

Figure 7.18. TAT images of the PIP joint of the left middle finger for R#2. (a)–(c) are cross-sectional TAT images of the joint with a spatial interval of 2mm between two adjacent slices. (d) is the ultrasound image of the joint.

figure 7.16, the TAT images of the four sections cover the completed PIP joint for H#1. No abnormalities were found in the TAT images of this joint.

R#1 (age = 69 years) suffers from rheumatoid arthritis and had pain on both sides of the PIP joint of the left middle finger. As shown in figure 7.17, the abnormal structures on the right side of the joint are clearly identified, and gradually weaken (see figure 7.17(a)–(d)). Some hypertrophic features of the left collateral ligament are roughly identified, as shown in figure 7.17(c) and (d). These two abnormalities coincide with the symptoms described by the patient. In addition, some abnormalities of the extensor tendon can be seen. R#2 (age = 70 years) suffers from rheumatoid arthritis, and the PIP joint of the right middle finger is abnormal. As shown in figure 7.18(a)–(c), the bone boundary is apparently not smooth, and the soft tissue cannot be distinguished clearly. From the ultrasound image of the same PIP joint for R# (figure 7.18(d)), we can see that the cortex of the joint is not smooth and the soft tissue is swollen.

To facilitate a comparison between the healthy and diseased groups, we place figure 7.16(a), 7.17(a) and 7.18(a) in a single figure as figure 7.19. Compared with the

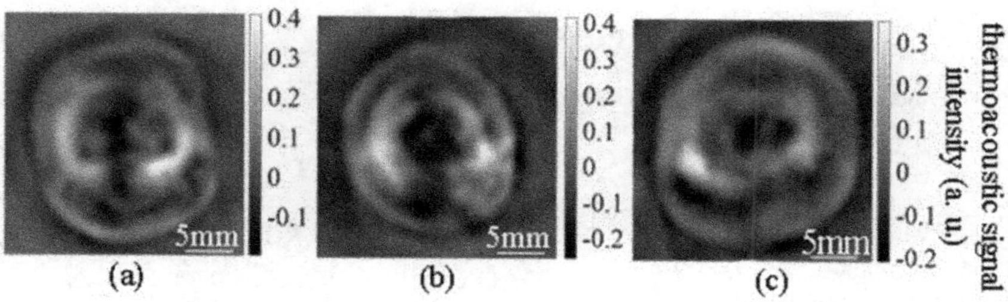

Figure 7.19. Thermoacoustic comparison between the healthy and diseased groups. (a) is the same as 7.16(a), (b) is the same as 7.17(a), and (c) is the same as 7.18(a).

healthy joint (figure 7.19(a)), the diseased joints show strong abnormalities (figure 7.19(b) and (c)). Specifically, R#1 has multiple local abnormalities, while R#2 has global abnormalities, which means that R#2 has more serious RA.

7.2 Brain imaging

Current imaging methods used to detect and diagnose brain diseases, like CT and MRI, are time-consuming, expensive and bulky. Thus they cannot be used in remote areas, or for monitoring brain injury over a long period of time. TAT, as a compact, mobile and inexpensive modality, can be applied to monitor a patient continuously in real time, either at the bedside or in an ambulance. In addition, TAT adds a significant advantage for brain imaging compared to the existing imaging methods to provide high resolution imaging of tissue conductivity. This unique ability would allow TAT to have a role in various electromagnetic (EM) brain simulations such as deep brain stimulation (DBS) and transcranial magnetic stimulation (TMS) to optimize the treatment of neurodisorders. Here we describe the applications of TAT to imaging of *in vivo* rat brain, and *ex vivo* and *in vivo* human brains.

7.2.1 *In vivo* rat brain

Reprinted from Zhao *et al* 2017.

Our experimental setup used for *in vivo* rat brain imaging is schematically shown in figure 7.20(a). In this TAT system, a custom-designed pulsed microwave generator (frequency: 3.0 GHz, peak power: 70 kW, pulse duration: 750 ns, repetition rate: 50 Hz) 18 was used to produce microwave pulses through a waveguide-fed pyramidal horn antenna (aperture size: 114×144 mm^2) to irradiate the rat head from the front (figure 7.20(b), coronal scanning) or from the top (figure 7.20(c), transverse scanning). A 5 MHz cylindrical focusing ultrasound transducer (V326, Olympus; diameter: 10 mm; focal length: 53 mm) rotated by a step motor detected the TA signal at 180 steps with a constant scanning step of 2° to cover a 2π-receiving angle. The signal detected was filtered (3 dB bandwidth: 500 kHz–30 MHz) and amplified by a low-noise pre-amplifier (Preamp2-D, US Ultratek, Inc., USA) with 60 dB. The signal was then sampled and averaged 50 times by data acquisition card controlled by a computer. The total time for data collection was 3 min. After a second-order Butterworth low-pass filter at 1.5 MHz to suppress noises, the TAT signals were used to reconstruct TAT images using the

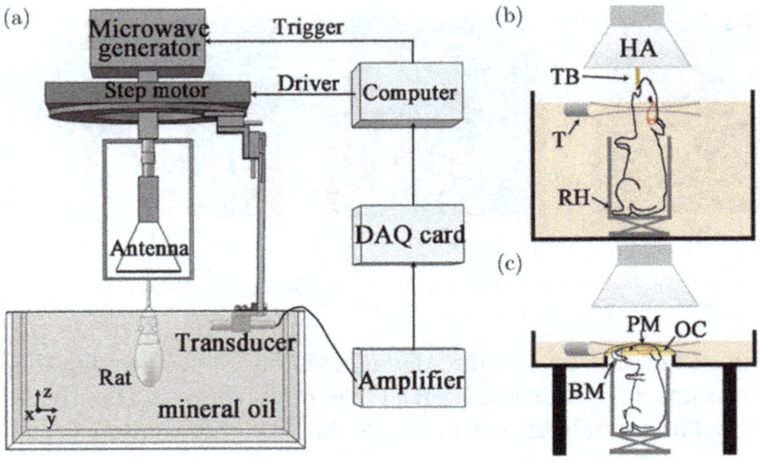

Figure 7.20. (a) Schematic of TAT system for imaging of rat brain. (b) and (c) Schematics showing the coronal and transverse scanning, respectively. RH: rat holder, PM: plastic membrane, OC: oil-based couplant, BM: breathing mask, TB: tooth bar, T: transducer and HA: waveguide-fed pyramidal horn antenna. Reprinted with permission from Zhao *et al* (2017).

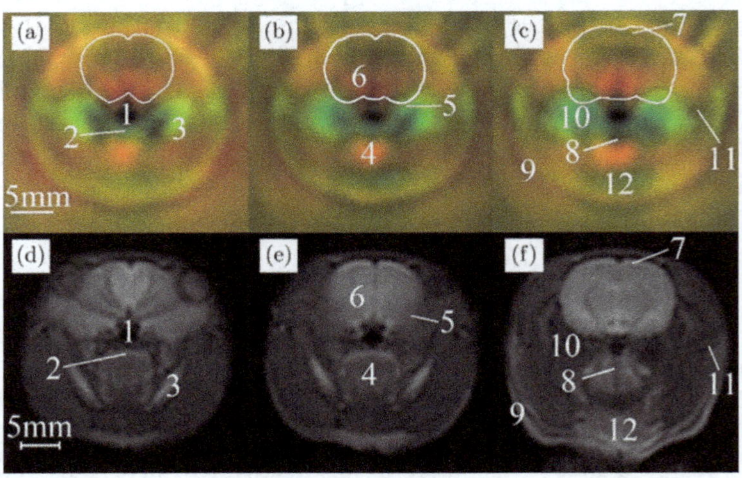

Figure 7.21. *In vivo* TAT (panels (a)–(c)) and 3T T2*-MRI (panels (d)–(f)) images of rat brain (n = 3) at different coronal sections. Anatomical structures are identified in these images according to the sectional anatomical atlas of Sprague-Dawley rat: 1: trachea, 2: palate bone, 3: mandible, 4: tongue, 5: temporal bone, 6: striatum, 7: neocortex, 8: larynx, 9: scalp, 10: middle ear, 11: zygomar and 12: gland. Reprinted with permission from Zhao *et al* (2017).

delay-and-sum algorithm. The actual averaged microwave power density at the surface of the rat brain is below 0.32 mW cm^{-2}, which is far below the safety standard (10 mW cm^{-2} at 3 GHz).

We obtained MRI images of a rat brain and conducted TAT imaging of the same rat brain (see figure 7.21). We found that the TAT images are comparable to the

MRI images to quite some extent and that numerous tissue structures seen on MRI are also revealed on TAT, including trachea, palate bone, mandible, tongue, temporal bone, striatum, neocortex, larynx, scalp, middle ear, zygomar and gland. These results suggest that TAT has great potential to be used in neuroscience studies. The spatial resolution of this system is estimated to be about 0.9 mm due to limitation by the pulse width of the microwave generator.

7.2.2 Phantom enclosed with *ex vivo* human skull

Reprinted with permission from Huang *et al* (2017).

According to the statistics published by the World Health Organization in 2010, almost 80% of all stroke cases are ischemic, while the rest are hemorrhagic. While it has a high rate of mortality, it is widely known that if an ischemic stroke patient could be treated by systemic thrombolysis within a time window of 4.5 h, the morbidity and mortality rate could be significantly reduced. Therefore, it is critical to timely detect an ischemic stroke and to distinguish it from a hemorrhage stroke before an established thrombolytic procedure is initiated. MRI and CT are currently used for stroke diagnosis. CT can identify a hemorrhage and detect early-stage acute ischemia. MRI can assess acute stroke and highlight the penumbra in particular. However, CT and MRI systems are quite bulky and often not mobile. TAT is relatively portable and mobile, making it uniquely suited for its use in an ambulance. Here we take an initial step to study the feasibility of TAT towards imaging the human brain using a tissue-mimicking phantom enclosed within a human skull. We conduct several phantom experiments to demonstrate that it is indeed possible to use TAT for noninvasive high contrast imaging of hemorrhagic stroke.

Figure 7.22 depicts the schematic of our TAT system. A 3.0 GHz pulsed microwave from a custom-designed magnetron generator (bandwidth: 50 MHz,

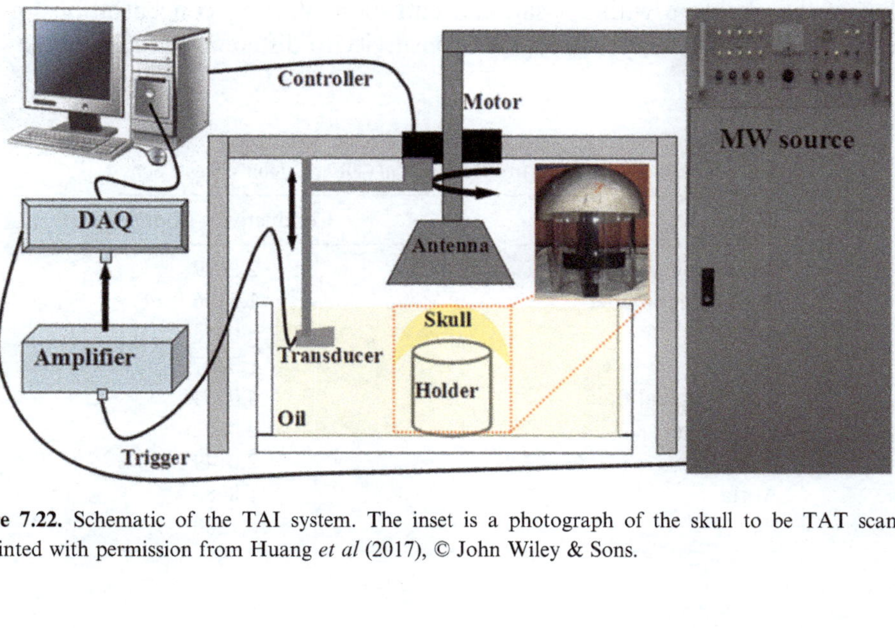

Figure 7.22. Schematic of the TAI system. The inset is a photograph of the skull to be TAT scanned. Reprinted with permission from Huang *et al* (2017), © John Wiley & Sons.

peak power: 70~100 kW, pulse duration: 0.75 μs, pulse repetition frequency: up to 1000 Hz) was coupled into the skull/phantom via a standard 10 dB gain horn antenna (114 × 144 mm^2) to generate thermoacoustic waves. While the peak power of our microwave source was high, the actual average microwave power density at the skull surface was only about 3.2 mW cm^{-2} when 10 Hz repetition frequency was used, which is far below the IEEE standard for safety levels (10 mW cm^{-2} at 3.0 GHz). For TA signal collection, the skull/phantom was immersed into a transformer oil filled tank for effective microwave/ultrasound signal transmission. An unfocused immersion transducer with (V323-SU, Olympus), mounted on a rotary stage (RSA 100, Beijing Zolix Instruments CO. LTD, China) and placed at 11.5 cm apart from the scanning center, was circularly scanned over 360° with a step size of 2° for TA signal collection. The transducer received TA signals were first amplified through a pre-amplifier (Pre-Amp 2D, US Ultratek, Inc., USA), then averaged 100 times with a data acquisition card (DAQ) (PCI4732, Chengdu vidts dynamic instrument company, LTD, Chengdu), and finally stored in a computer for subsequent image reconstruction. Synchronization and control of the hardware components were realized by a Labview (National Instruments Corporation, Austin, TX) program. Image reconstruction was performed using the delay-and-sum algorithm created by MATLAB (Mathworks Inc., Natic, MA).

Table 7.2. indicates that the conductivity contrast between blood and gray/white matter is up to 2 at 3 GHz. When a hemorrhagic stroke occurs, blood will flux to gray white matter, inducing a significant contrast for thermoacoustic imaging.

A human adult skull (roughly: 180 × 140 mm^2) coupled with agar powder (10%) mixed with different concentrations of salt were used to mimic brain tissue. The salt concentrations used in our experiments (1%, 2%, 3% and 4%) gave a conductivity of the object of 1.80 S m^{-1}, 3.20 S m^{-1}, 4.36 S m^{-1} and 6.07 S m^{-1}, respectively. For all the experiments, the background phantom (serving as 'normal brain tissue') contained 1% salt concentration. From table 7.2, the conductivity of blood is close to that of the phantom with 2% salt concentration. Various concentrations of salt were used in the target(s) to study TAT sensitivity to different contrast levels.

Table 7.2. Conductivity property of major human brain tissues at 3 GHz. Reproduced with permission from Huang *et al* (2017), © John Wiley & Sons.

Material	Conductivity (S m^{-1})
Brain gray matter	2.2189
Brain white matter	1.5106
Blood	3.0498
Nerve	1.3297
Cerebrospinal fluid	4.0054
Cerebellum	2.4822
Dura	2.0149
Aorta	1.8080
Fat	0.1300

The background phantom with 1% salt concentration was first heated and then poured into the skull. After solidification, a brain-shaped phantom was made and the background phantom was separated from the skull. Several holes were drilled in the upper surface of the background phantom, into which targets containing higher salt concentration were inserted to mimic hemorrhagic stroke. Finally, the background phantom was covered again by the skull for TAT imaging.

7.2.2.1 A single target

In the first experiment, a rectangular target (30 × 11 mm^2) containing 2% salt concentration (σ = 3.20 S m^{-1}) was used to simulate a single hemorrhagic spot. Figure 7.23(a) shows a photograph of the phantom where the target (in black) was embedded in the background normal 'brain tissue' (in white). During TA data collection, the phantom was overlaid by the human skull, as indicated in figure 7.22. Figure 7.23(b) is the reconstructed TA image obtained using the delay-and-sum algorithm. It is seen that both the target and skull features were clearly recovered.

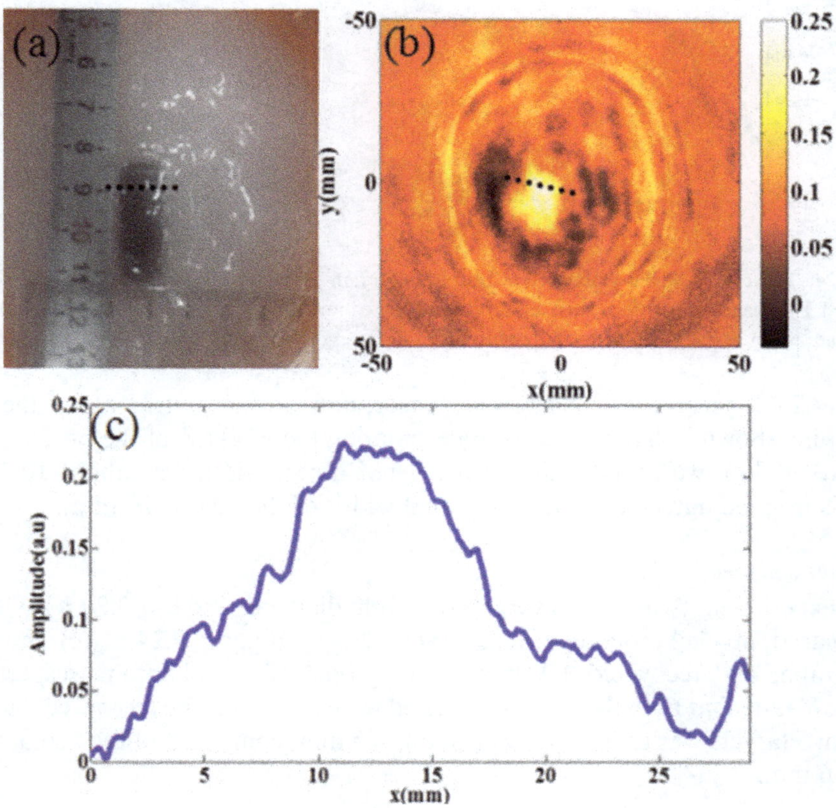

Figure 7.23. TAI of a single target embedded in background normal brain tissue. (a) Photograph of the target-containing phantom. (b) Recovered TA image when the phantom was overlaid by the human skull. (c) Reconstructed microwave absorption profile along the dark dashed line shown in (a) and (b). Reprinted with permission from Huang *et al* (2017), © John Wiley & Sons.

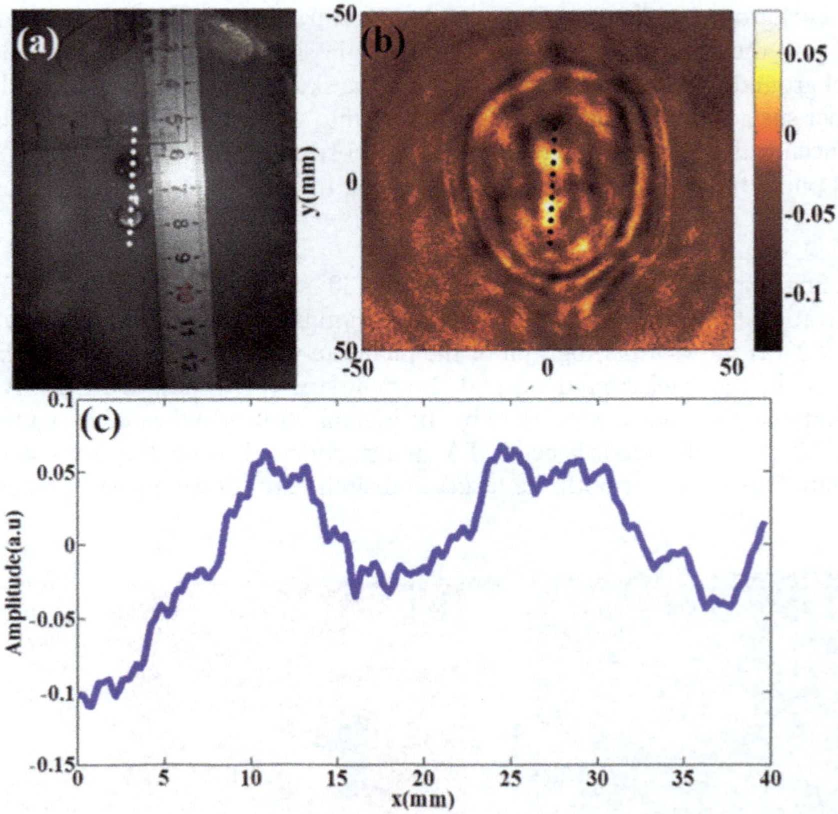

Figure 7.24. TAI of two targets embedded in background brain tissue. (a) Photograph of the phantom. (b) Recovered TA image of the phantom/skull. (c) Reconstructed microwave absorption profile along the dark dashed line shown in (b). Reprinted with permission from Huang *et al* (2017), © John Wiley & Sons.

Figure 7.23(c) presents the microwave absorption profile plotted along the dark dashed line shown in figure 7.23(b). By estimating the FWHM of the profile shown in figure 7.23(c), we found that the recovered object width was about 10.5 mm, which is in good agreement with the actual width of the target (11 mm).

7.2.2.2 Two targets

In this experiment, two circular targets (6 mm in diameter and $\sigma = 3.20$ S m^{-1} each) were placed in background normal 'brain tissue'. Figures 7.24(a)–(c) show the photograph, and recovered TA image and profile of the phantom, respectively. Again, we note that both the targets and skull were revealed. The recovered diameter of the two targets was estimated to be about 5.5 mm, compared to the actual target size of 6 mm.

7.2.2.3 Three targets

Here we embedded three targets with 2%, 3% and 4% salt concentration in the background phantom, as shown in figures 7.25(a) and (b). Figure 7.25(c) gives the

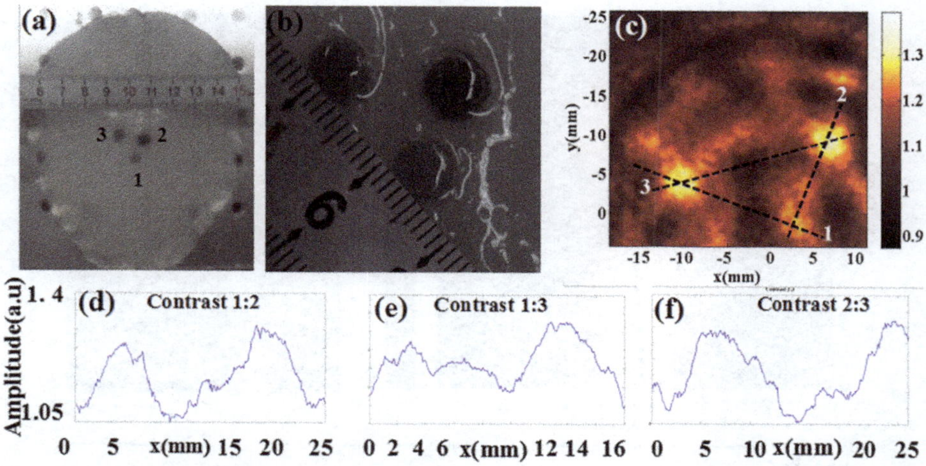

Figure 7.25. TAI of three targets (1, 2 and 3) embedded in background normal brain tissue. (a) Photograph of the phantom. (b) Close-up view of the phantom. (c) Recovered TA image. (d)–(f) Reconstructed microwave absorption profiles along the dark dashed lines 1–3, 1–2 and 2–3 shown in (a). Reprinted with permission from Huang *et al* (2017), © John Wiley & Sons.

reconstructed TA image when the phantom was covered by the human skull. Immediately we noted that the relative position and shape of the three targets were clearly recovered, and that targets 2 and 3 were better recovered relative to target 1 due to their larger conductivity contrast. Figures 7.25(d)–(f) present the microwave absorption profiles plotted along the three dark dashed lines (1–3, 1–2 and 2–3) shown in figure 7.25(c). The TA recovered diameters of targets 1, 2 and 3 were about 3.5, 4.0 and 4.5 mm, respectively, which matched well with the actual diameter of the targets (4 mm).

7.2.2.4 Spatial resolution

To estimate the spatial resolution of TAT for hemorrhagic stroke detection, two copper wires with diameters of 100 μm were inserted into the background phantom at a distance of 2 mm, as indicated in figure 7.26(a). The recovered TA image of the two copper wires was shown in figure 7.26(b). To calculate the spatial resolution of this system, the TA signal profile along the dark dashed line (figure 7.26(b)) is given in figure 7.26(c). According to the Rayleigh criterion (R), the 40.5% amplitude line in figure 7.26(c) intercepts the profile at points A, B, C and D. Thus the spatial resolution can be approximated as $R = 0.5 \times (|AB| + |CD|) - d$, where d is the diameter of the copper wire; hence the spatial resolution is estimated to be about 0.9 mm. The spatial resolution is primarily limited by the pulse width of the microwave generator.

In summary, we have presented a study representing a significant step toward *in vivo* thermoacoustic imaging of hemorrhage stroke. While the results presented are encouraging, there are still improvements needed before we can conduct such *in vivo* imaging. First, the frequency of microwaves for ultrasound excitation needs to be optimized. For example, as hemorrhage stroke is our goal, a microwave

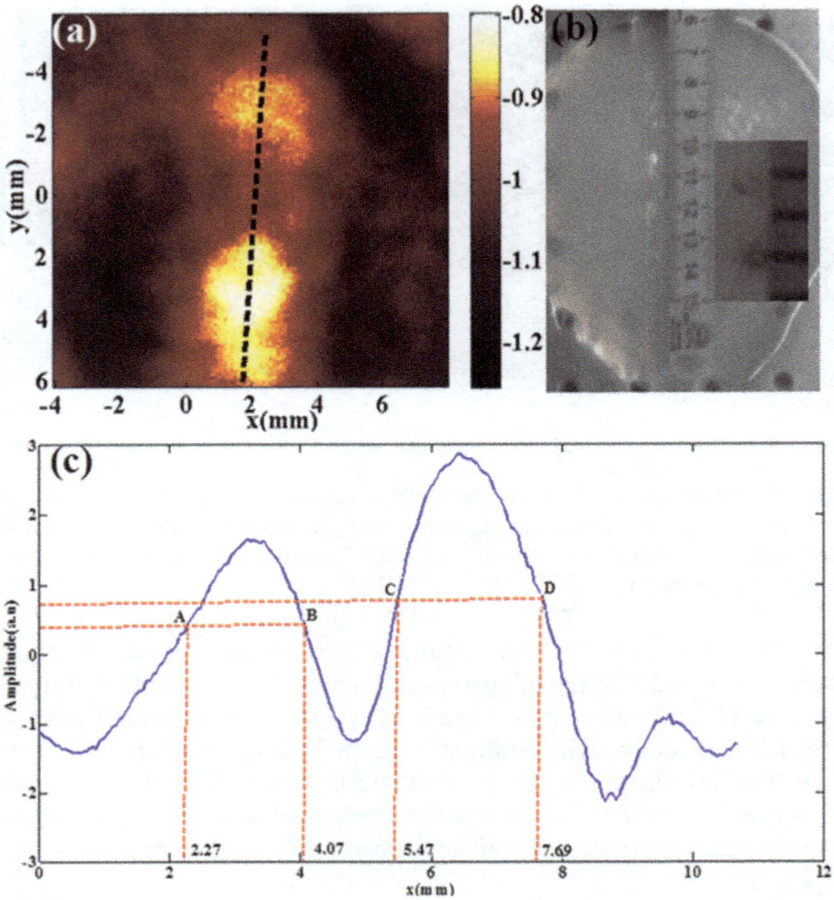

Figure 7.26. TAI of two copper wires embedded in the background phantom for system spatial resolution evaluation. (a) Recovered TA image. (b) Photograph of the phantom. (c) Reconstructed microwave absorption profile along the dark dashed line shown in (a). Reprinted with permission from Huang *et al* (2017), © John Wiley & Sons.

frequency that is most sensitive to blood is preferred. In addition, for clinical application, a variety of bio-effects and safety issues must be carefully considered. Finally, an antenna system which can provide a homogeneous energy distribution in the brain is desired. To achieve a high temporal resolution, a multiple channel DAQ system is currently under investigation in our lab. Nonetheless, this study has demonstrated the potential role that TAT may have in detecting hemorrhage stroke *in vivo*.

7.2.3 *In vivo* human brain

We also conducted a first-in-human study to image a healthy human brain using a thermoacoustic imager schematically shown in figure 7.27. A 3.0 GHz pulsed microwave from a custom-designed microwave generator was coupled into the brain

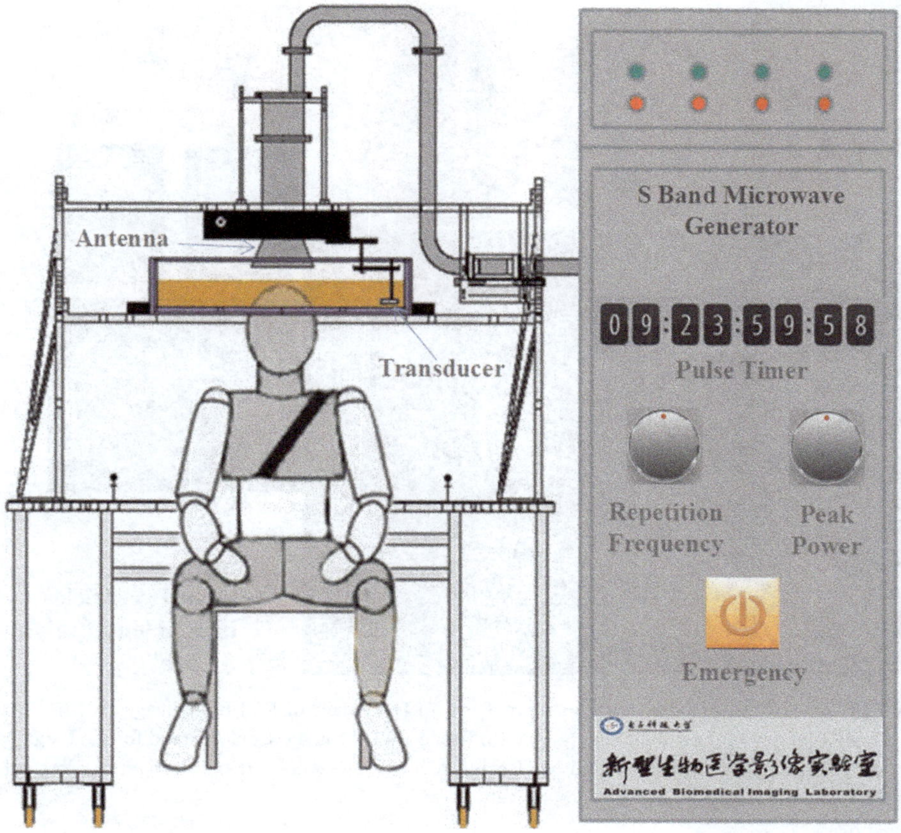

Figure 7.27. Experimental setup for thermoacoustic brain imaging. An S-band microwave generator transmitted microwaves into the brain via a conical horn antenna for acoustic signal evoking. An immersed transducer circularly scans the scene for data collection. Transformer oil (yellow) was used for microwave and ultrasound signals coupling.

via a horn antenna to generate thermoacoustic waves. Unlike most TAT systems, which use rectangular horn antenna or waveguide to transmit the microwaves, the radiator used in this study employed a conical horn antenna (diameter = 190 mm). This modification offered a sufficient radiation area for whole brain imaging with improved energy uniformity compared to conventional TAT implementations. An unfocused immersion transducer with a central frequency of 2.25 MHz mounted on a rotary stage was used for signal receiving. We imaged a volunteer's brain to investigate the feasibility of this TAT system.

We obtained five slices of TAT images from the volunteer's brain. Figure 7.28 shows three typical TA recovered slices compared with the corresponding T1 MRI images of the same brain. The cerebral spinal fluid filled lateral ventricle is identified by TAT as it has a significant contrast in conductivity compared with surrounding white matter ($\sigma = 4.0$ S m^{-1} vs. $\sigma = 1.5$ S m^{-1}). The size of the lateral ventricle is relatively larger than other tissues in the brain, and it looks like a 'butterfly', which is

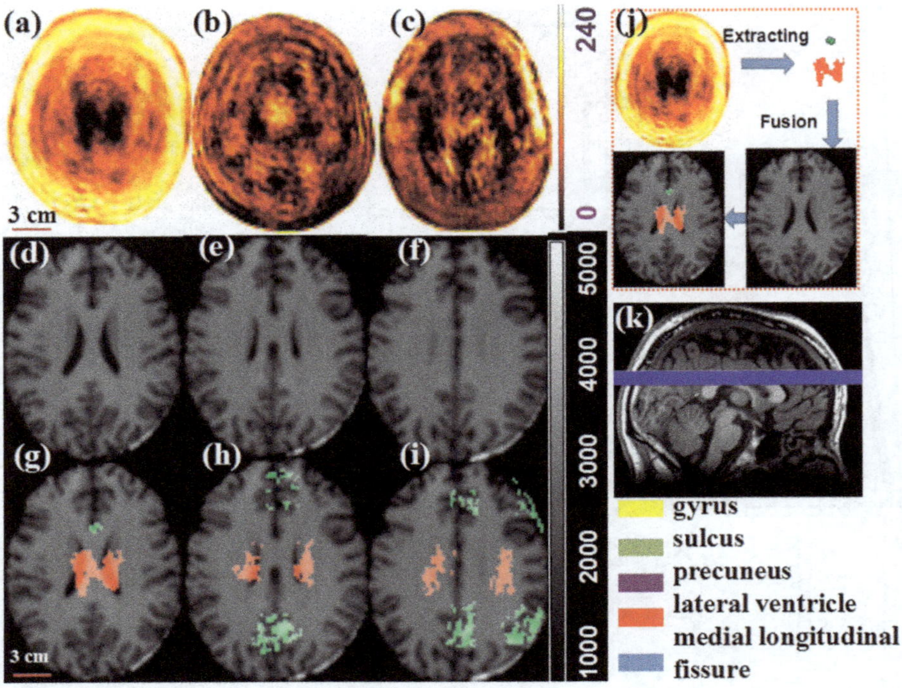

Figure 7.28. *In vivo* TAT imaging of a human brain. (a)–(c) Three slices of TAT brain images. (d)–(f) 2D axial brain T1 MRI images of the same brain. (g) and (h) Fused TAT-T1 images, colors stand for TAT signals. (j) Schematic of image fusion. (k) TAT and MRI scanned slices. The color bar on the right side present the relative TAT and MRI signal intensity, respectively.

clearly revealed in the TA images (figures 7.28(a)–(c)). From figure 7.28(j), some remarkable features of the TA image are extracted from different ROIs (regions of interest), and are then overlayed with the corresponding T1 images (figures 7.28(d)–(f)). In figures 7.28(g)–(i), the areas in red represent the structure of the 'butterfly' shaped lateral ventricle.

Based on the brain anatomy, the sulcus and gyrus are surrounded by cerebrospinal fluid., and clearly imaged by TAT, as shown by the areas in green and yellow in figures 7.28(g)–(i). While the spatial resolution and contrast of this TAT imager would allow for imaging most of the brain structures, we note that only parts of these structures are revealed (figures 7.28(g)–(i)). This is primarily due to the fact that the TAT imaging is strongly dependent upon the polarization angle of the electric field (E-field) and the morphology of tissue—the structures with their long axis parallel to the E-field generate the strongest TA signals. However, we believe that more brain tissue types could be resolved by TAT if a microwave source with optimized orientation of E-field polarization is used.

7.3 Imaging of thyroid

The thyroid gland is the largest endocrine gland in the human body. It controls the synthesis of thyroid hormones to maintain normal metabolism of the body, and plays a vital role in the metabolism, growth and maturity of the nervous system. According to the American Cancer Society, the incidence of thyroid cancer in the United States (US) increased at a rate of 5% per year since 2003 (Enewold *et al* 2009). Epidemiologists believe that by 2030, thyroid cancer will become the fourth most prevalent cancer in the US (Rahib *et al* 2014, Vecchia *et al* 2015), and the prevalence of thyroid nodules is more than 60% (Guth *et al* 2009, Gharib *et al* 2016). All the malignant cases found in thyroid nodules account for about 10%, mainly composed of differentiated thyroid cancer, including papillary thyroid cancer and follicular cancer (Cooper *et al* 2006). The key to the treatment of thyroid nodules is the early and accurate detection of thyroid cancer (Hegedüs 2004).

Current imaging methods for examining thyroid gland include ultrasound, CT, MRI, radionuclide imaging, and fine needle aspiration biopsy under image guidance. Although these examination methods have their own advantages, they have shortcomings. For example, while ultrasound is the most widely used method for thyroid examination, it is highly dependent on the physician's skills and cannot independently distinguish the benign and malignant thyroid nodules. MRI's specificity, sensitivity and accuracy are higher than ultrasound, but it is costly and not suitable for long-term monitoring. Image-guided fine needle aspiration biopsy is the gold standard for the diagnosis of thyroid nodules, but it is invasive. Here we aim to examine the feasibility of thermoacoustic tomography (TAT) to image the human thyroid gland.

7.3.1 Thermoacoustic imaging system

The TAT system used to image the thyroid is schematically shown in figure 7.29(a). It is mainly composed of a microwave source, a data acquisition system and an image reconstruction module. The microwave source has a center frequency of 3.0 GHz, a pulse width of 0.75 μs, and a peak power of 70 kW. Microwave pulses are delivered to the object through a 1.5 m long coaxial cable coupled with an open-ended waveguide, which is attached to a flexible transducer array/thyroid interface with an angle of 45°. The flexible transducer array has a total of 128 elements with a center frequency of 2.25 MHz and a bandwidth of 70% (Japan probe, JAPAN) (figure 7.29(b)). The interface has a radius of $R = 141$ mm, and covers 160.5° along the neck (figure 7.29(c)). A thin plastic bag containing mineral oil is placed between the interface and the skin. In addition, ultrasonic gel is applied to the skin to further optimize the ultrasound transmission. TA signals collected by the array are amplified by pre-amplifiers, and digitized by two 32-channel data acquisition cards (5752b, National Instruments, USA). The entire data acquisition process is controlled by Labview programming, and the image reconstruction is performed by the delay-and-sum method. A complete data acquisition and image reconstruction process takes about 5 s.

Thyroid glands of three volunteers (one male, two females, average age = 23 years old) are examined. The imaging plane includes the left and right lobes of the thyroid gland (figure 7.29(d)). For comparison, a commercial clinical-scale ultrasound system (iNSIGHT 37C, Saset Healthcare, Inc.) is used to image the same thyroid glands.

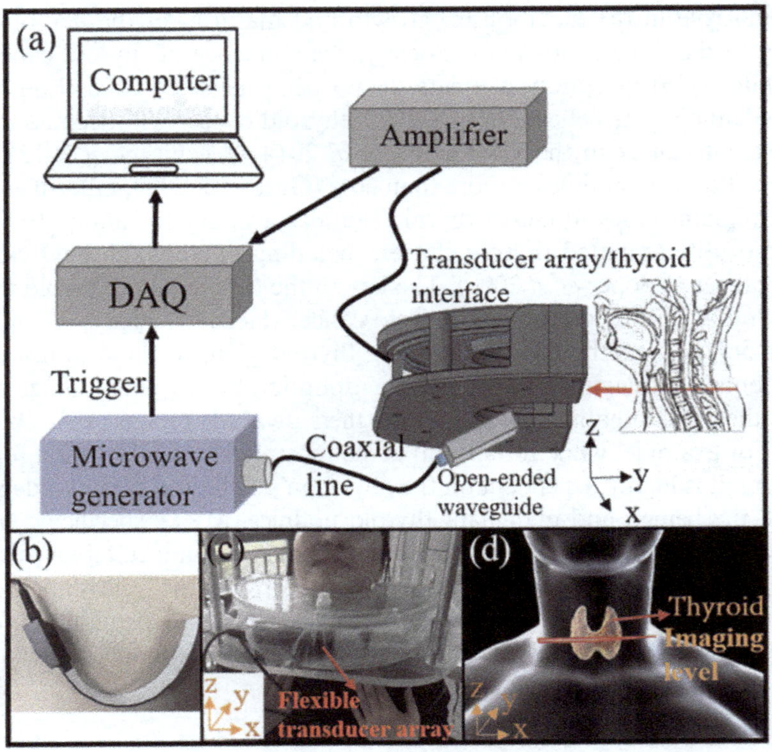

Figure 7.29. (a) Schematic of the thermoacoustic imaging for thyroid imaging. (b) Photograph of the flexible transducer array. (c) Photograph of the transducer array/thyroid interface. (d) Schematic of the imaging plane for TAT and ultrasound. Reprinted with permission from Wang *et al* (2019).

7.3.2 Results and discussion

Figure 7.30 presents TAT (figures 7.30(d) and (e)) and ultrasound (figures 7.30(a)–(c)) images for volunteer A. Figure 7.30(a) shows the frontal ultrasound image showing the anatomical structures including thyroid isthmus and trachea, while figures 7.30(b) and (c) are the ultrasound images of the left and right lobes, respectively, showing the anatomical features including the trachea, thyroid and carotid artery. From figure 7.30(d), in comparison with the corresponding ultrasound image, the TAT image clearly reveals the skin boundary as well as the trachea and thyroid (including the isthmus). In addition, the boundary of the esophagus is identified.

To further verify the TAT images for volunteer A, we calculated the tracheal diameter, the lateral width of the left thyroid, the longitudinal length of the left thyroid, the lateral width of the right thyroid and the longitudinal length of the right thyroid, and compare these parameters with those measured by ultrasound. The orange lines in figures 7.30(a)–(c) indicate the same positions as the red lines segment in figure 7.30(e). Along these orange and red lines, we plot the ultrasound (top) and TAT (bottom) image profiles in figure 7.31 where the sizes of different tissue

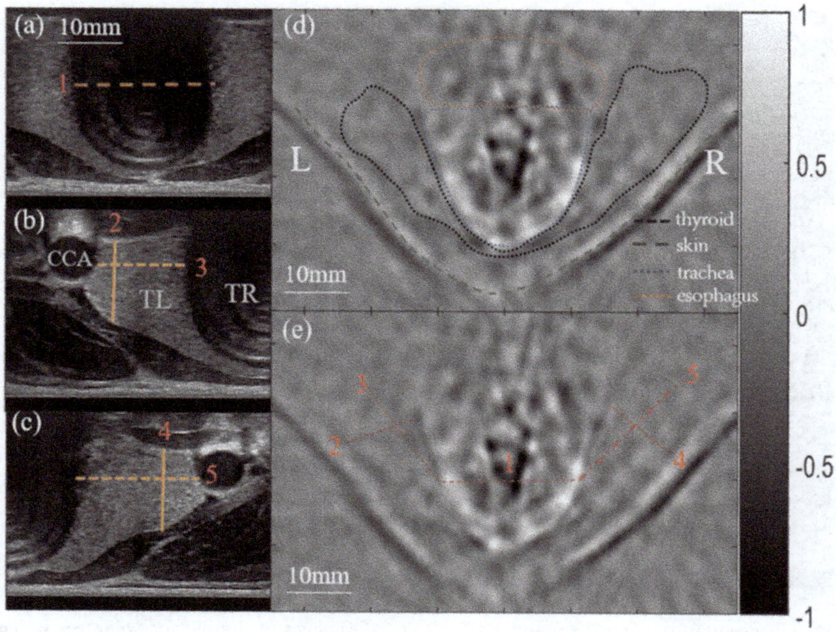

Figure 7.30. Ultrasound (a), (b) and (c) and TAT (d) and (e) images of thyroid for volunteer A. The areas highlighted by different colors in (d) indicate different tissue types. The red lines in (e) mark the same position as the orange lines in (a), (b), and (c) for further analysis given in figure 7.31. l: left; R: right; CCA: common carotid artery; TL: thyroid; TR: trachea; ES: esophagus. The color bar on the right indicates the relative intensity of the thermoacoustic signal. Reprinted with permission from Wang *et al* (2019).

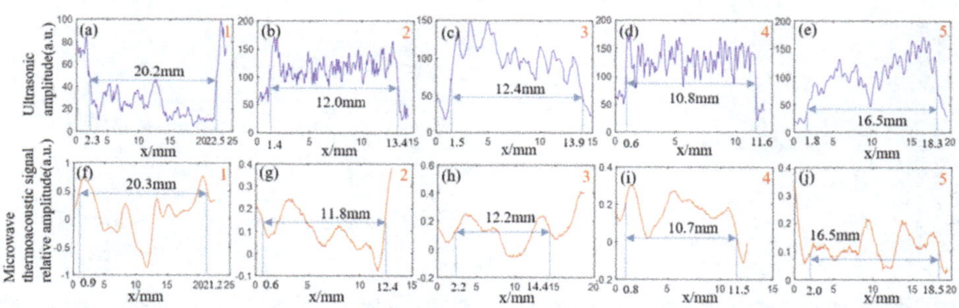

Figure 7.31. Volunteer A: Ultrasound (top) and TAT (bottom) image profiles along the orange and red lines shown in figures 7.30(a)–(c) and figure 7.30(e), respectively. The size of the tracheal (a), (f), the lateral width of the left thyroid lobe (b), (g), the longitudinal length of the left thyroid lobe (c), (h), the lateral width of the right thyroid lobe (d), (i), and the longitudinal length of the right thyroid (e), (j). Reprinted with permission from Wang *et al* (2019).

structures are also given, which are calculated using the FWHM of the profiles. We immediately note that these sizes measured by TAT and ultrasound match very well. TAT and ultrasound images along their image profiles for volunteers B and C are given in figures 7.32 and 7.33, and figures 7.34 and 7.35, respectively. We see that the TAT image quality and the comparison with the ultrasound for volunteers B and C are similar to those for volunteer A.

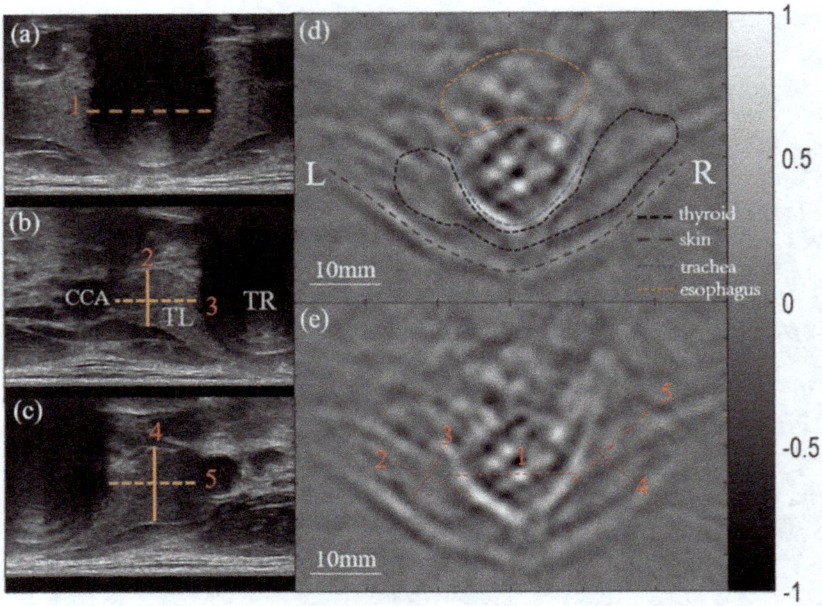

Figure 7.32. Ultrasound (a), (b) and (c) and TAT (d) and (e) images of thyroid for volunteer B. The areas highlighted by different colors in (d) indicate different tissue types. The red lines in (e) mark the same position as the orange lines in (a), (b), and (c) for further analysis given in figure 7.31. L: left; R: right; CCA: common carotid artery; TL: thyroid; TR: trachea; ES: esophagus. The color bar on the right indicates the relative intensity of the thermoacoustic signal. Reprinted with permission from Wang *et al* (2019).

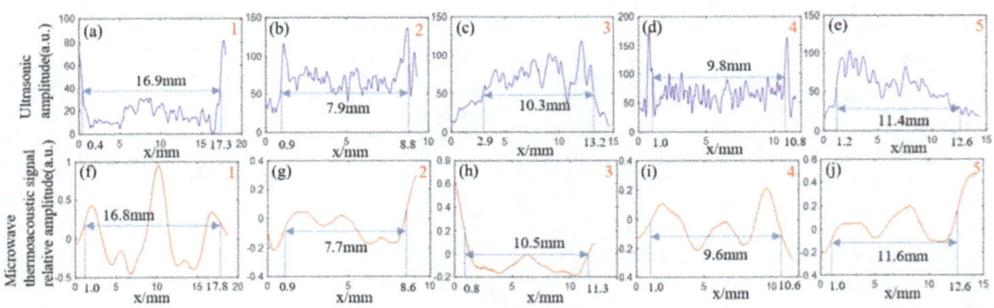

Figure 7.33. Volunteer B: Ultrasound (top) and TAT (bottom) image profiles along the orange and red lines shown in figures 7.30(a)–(c) and (e), respectively. The size of the tracheal (a), (f), the lateral width of the left thyroid lobe (b), (g), the longitudinal length of the left thyroid lobe (c), (h), the lateral width of the right thyroid lobe (d), (i), and the longitudinal length of the right thyroid (e), (j). Reprinted with permission from Wang *et al* (2019).

7.4 Liver imaging

Microwave ablation (MWA) is a current clinical tool for treating cancers of the liver, kidney, lung, breast and adrenal gland by thermally ablating the lesions (Wright *et al* 2005, Simon *et al* 2005). Unfortunately, due to the lack of guidance, under- or over-treatment of a lesion by MWA has been a major cause of procedural failure, resulting in repeated treatments (Vogl *et al* 2017). Thus, an accurate and

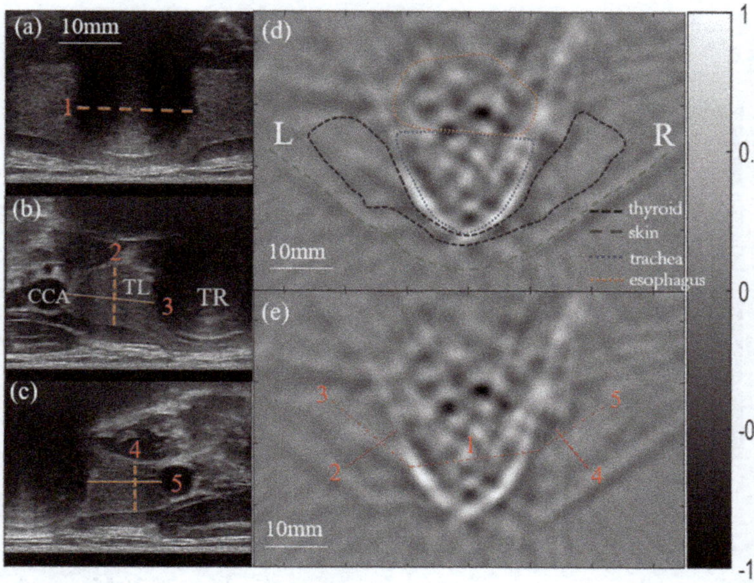

Figure 7.34. Ultrasound (a), (b) and (c) and TAT (d) and (e) images of thyroid for volunteer C. The areas highlighted by different colors in (d) indicate different tissue types. The red lines in (e) mark the same position as the orange lines in (a), (b), and (c) for further analysis given in figure 7.31. L: left; R: right; CCA: common carotid artery; TL: thyroid; TR: trachea; ES: esophagus. The color bar on the right indicates the relative intensity of the thermoacoustic signal. Reprinted with permission from Wang *et al* (2019).

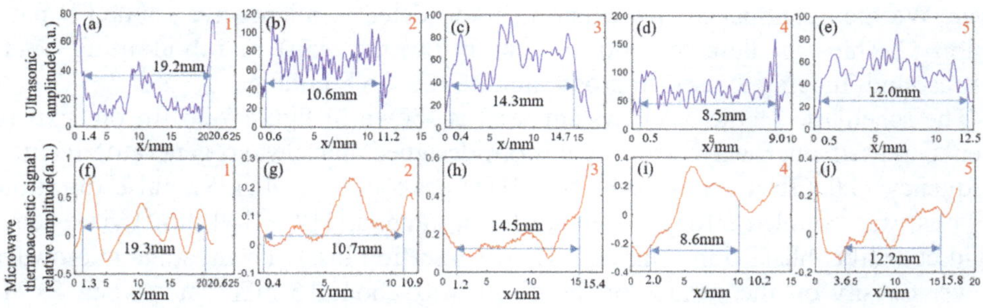

Figure 7.35. Volunteer C: Ultrasound (top) and TAT (bottom) image profiles along the orange and red lines shown in figures 7.30(a)–(c) and (e), respectively. The size of the tracheal (a), (f), the lateral width of the left thyroid lobe (b), (g), the longitudinal length of the left thyroid lobe (c), (h), the lateral width of the right thyroid lobe (d), (i), and the longitudinal length of the right thyroid (e), (j). Reprinted with permission from Wang *et al* (2019).

reliable imaging technique that can assess MWA timely during the procedure is essential to determine the efficacy of therapy. In this regard, ultrasound (US), x-ray computed tomography (CT), and magnetic resonance imaging (MRI) have been explored; however, it is hard for these imaging techniques to evaluate lesion formation during the procedure due to their limited temporal resolution (for CT and MRI) or low contrast (for US) (Zhang *et al* 2018). Numerous studies have shown that dielectric properties of lesion during an MWA procedure change

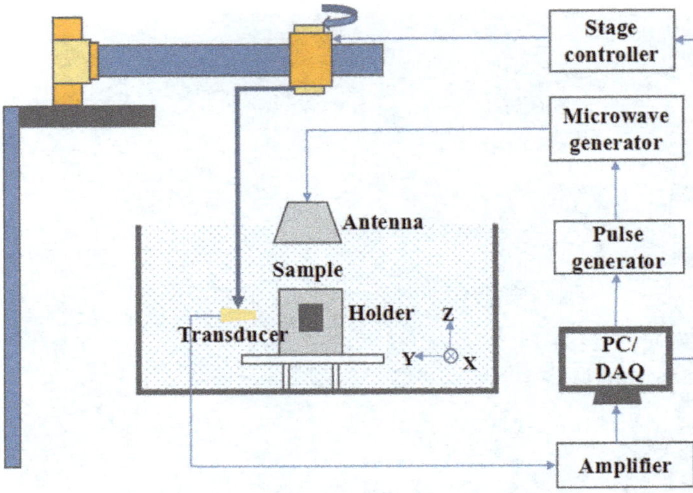

Figure 7.36. Schematic of TAI experimental setup.

significantly due to decrease in tissue water content (Endo *et al* 2015) and increase in tissue temperature (Lazebnik *et al* 2006). This change of tissue dielectric properties can induce a microwave absorption contrast between normal and ablated tissues, which can be measured by TAT. In this section, we describe the use of TAT to noninvasively evaluate hepatic microwave ablation. The concept is demonstrated first by thermoacoustically imaging microwave ablated lesion in *ex vivo* porcine liver. We then conduct *in vivo* experiments to detect a microwave ablated hepatic lesion (22 mm in diameter and 10 mm below the skin) in rabbit using TAT. Ultrasound imaging is used to cross-validate the TAT findings.

The schematic of the TAT system used is shown in figure 7.36. In our experiments, pulsed microwave from a custom-designed microwave generator (central frequency: 3.0 GHz, bandwidth: 50 MHz, peak power: 70 kW, pulse duration: 0.75 μs) was coupled into a pyramidal horn antenna (114 × 144 mm^2) via a semi-rigid coaxial cable (1.5 m long with 1.2 dB insertion loss). The average microwave power density on the surface of the object was about 15 mW cm^{-2} when 50 Hz repetition frequency was used, which was below the IEEE standard for safety levels (20 mW cm^{-2} at 3.0 GHz). An immersion transducer with a central frequency of 2.25 MHz (V323-SU, Olympus), which was mounted on a rotary stage (RSA 100, Beijing Zolix Instruments Co. Ltd, China), was circularly scanned over 360° and 220° for *ex vivo* and *in vivo* experiment, respectively, with a step size of 2° for TA signal detection. For effective microwave/ultrasound signal coupling, both the object and the transducer were immersed into a transformer oil filled tank. The TA signals received by the transducer were amplified through a homemade amplifier, then averaged 50 times with a data acquisition card, and finally stored in a computer for image reconstruction. The total experimental time for one frame of image was 2 min; image reconstruction was performed utilizing the delay-and-sum algorithm.

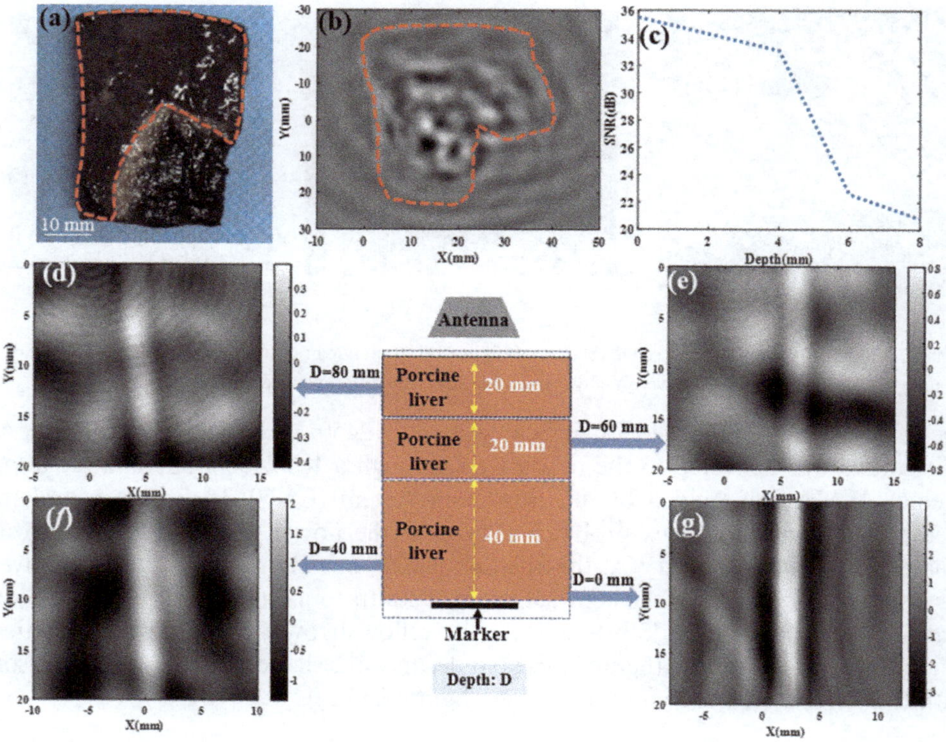

Figure 7.37. Photograph (a) and TAT image of a piece of *ex vivo* porcine liver having a soldering iron induced lesion in the right corner, (c) SNR versus imaging depth. (d)–(g) TAI recovered images by adding 80, 60, 40 and 0 mm porcine liver to the top of a 3 mm diameter tube containing soybean sauce.

For the *ex vivo* study, a fresh porcine liver was obtained from a local slaughter house. A soldering iron was used to simulate MWA to produce an approximately $8 \times 10 \times 5$ mm^3 thermal lesion in the porcine liver (right corner in figure 7.37(a) where the normal tissue is outlined by a red dashed line). Figure 7.37(b) presents the TAT recovered image of the liver where the boundary of the normal tissue is also indicated with a red dashed line. Here it can be seen that the TA signal from the lesion area was significantly smaller compared to that from the normal tissue, resulting in a clear 'blank' region in the right corner of the liver. To evaluate the ability of imaging depth, fresh porcine livers with different thicknesses were added to the top of a 3 mm diameter tube containing soybean sauce. Figures 7.37(d)–(g) show the TAT recovered images by adding 80, 60, 40 and 0 mm thick porcine liver to the top of the tube, respectively. We note that the tube is clearly seen when the thickness is 80 mm (figure 7.37(e)). As the imaging depth increased, the SNR decreased from 36 to 21 dB, as displayed in figure 7.37(c).

In vivo experiments were conducted using an adult New Zealand male rabbit (weight: 2 kg). Before the experiment, the fur on the abdomen of the rabbit was shaven. A dose of 40 mg kg^{-1} sodium pentobarbital was administered to anesthetize the rabbit via an ear vein before the MWA and TAI procedures. A holder was used to

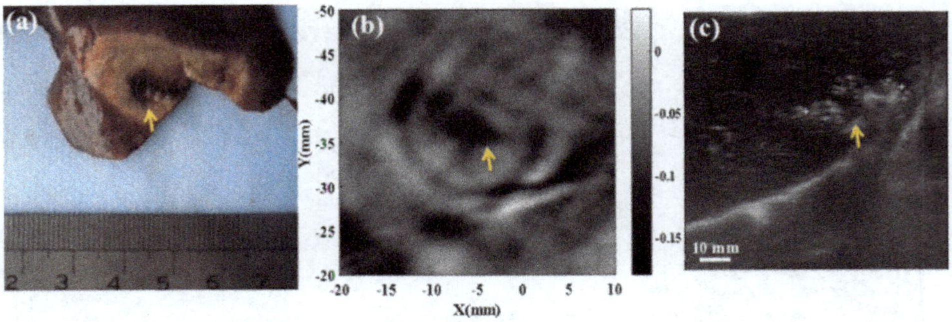

Figure 7.38. Photograph of the resected ablated rabbit liver after imaging (a), and *in vivo* TAT (b) and CE-US (c) images of the ablated rabbit liver. Yellow arrows indicate the microwave ablated lesion.

keep the rabbit immobilized. A clinical system at 2450 MHz was used for MWA. Microwave was delivered to the rabbit liver through a KY2450A antenna (ablation needle). WMA was guided by an ultrasound system (CX50, Philips, Amsterdam, Netherlands) with a convex probe (5–1). Under the power of 50 W, the liver was ablated for 3 min. After MWA, the ablation needle was inserted into the rabbit liver for lesion localization, see the contrast-enhanced ultrasound (CE-US) (figure 7.38(c)) and TAT images (figure 7.38(b)), indicated by yellow arrows. The microwave ablated lesion was clearly detected (figure 7.38(b)) in terms of its shape and size in comparison with the ultrasound image and pathology (figure 7.38(a)).

7.5 Vascular imaging

Blood vessels are an important part of the body, and their health affects the whole body's physiological function. It is known that blood temperature, blood content, blood oxygenation, blood vessel occlusion, and myocardial ischemia affect tissue dielectric properties, which offers a great contrast for TAT. Here we demonstrate the feasibility of TAT for vascular imaging in humans (reprinted from Zheng *et al* 2018).

In this study, a homemade microwave generator (700 ns pulse width, 3.0 GHz frequency, 70 kW peak power) was used as the excitation source. The thermoacoustic signals were acquired through a 128-element linear array transducer (8.5 MHz center frequency, SH7L38, SASET. Inc., China), and the TAT system used is schematically shown in figure 7.39, which contained a home-made 128-channel amplifier and a 64-channel acquisition system (5752B, NI. Inc., USA) for signal collection. To improve the quality of the signals, 50 times averaging was adopted, leading to a data acquisition time of ~2 s. Ultrasound images were collected through an ultrasound module using the same 128-element linear array transducer. Thus, both the TAT and ultrasound images can be precisely co-registered. It should be added that like in ultrasound imaging (US) Hilbert transform was also used in TAT image reconstruction. In the experiments, the objects being imaged were completely immersed in mineral oil for optimal coupling for both microwave and ultrasound deliveries. In particular, efforts were made to obtain best polarization direction of antenna to optimize the deposition of microwave energy in tissue (and blood vessels).

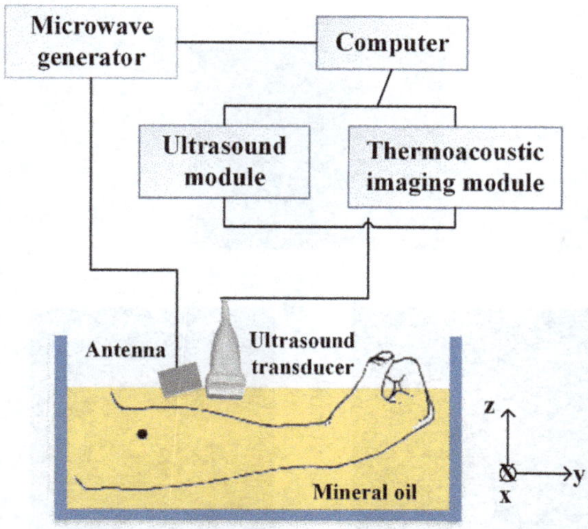

Figure 7.39. Schematic of the experimental setup. Reprinted from Zheng *et al* (2018), with the permission of AIP Publishing.

To demonstrate the ability of *in vivo* imaging blood vessels, the forearms of two volunteers were scanned. The transducer was placed about 1 cm away from the arm to minimize the influence of microwave to the transducer. Figure 7.40(a) shows the photograph of the forearm for one subject, and the blood vessels are indicated by a red square with a black dashed line representing the imaging plane. Figures 7.40(b) and (d)–(e), respectively, show the cross-sectional ultrasound, thermoacoustic, and overlaid TAT/US images for a representative subject. In the thermoacoustic image (figure 7.40(d)), there is a round spot in the center of the image (indicated by the red circle), which is confirmed to be a blood vessel (see the red circle in the corresponding ultrasound image). To confirm this, Doppler US was performed and the image is given in figure 7.40(c). We found that the distance from the blood vessel to the skin was about 3.36 mm from the TA image (figure 7.40(d)), which is also in good agreement with the ultrasound (figure 7.40(b)). The normalized TA and US profiles along a cut line through the center of the blood vessel are plotted in figure 7.40(f), from which the size of the recovered blood vessel was measured to be 3.36, and 2.90 mm by TAT and US, respectively. The spectrogram of thermoacoustic signals is also displayed in figure 7.40(g) for subsequent analysis. As shown in figure 7.40(g), the central frequency of the thermoacoustic signals is less than 1 MHz, suggesting that the spatial resolution of this system is ~1 mm according to the diffraction limit.

We also obtained sagittal-sectional images of blood vessels from another volunteer. Figure 7.41(a)–(d) presents the photograph, and TAT, US and overlaid TAT/US images. In figure 7.41(a), a red square highlights the blood vessel's location and a black dashed line indicates the imaging plane. From the TA (figure 7.41(b)) and US (figure 7.41(c)) images, the recovered size of the blood vessel was found to be 4.7 and 5.6 mm by TAI and US, respectively. We also note that the contrast of the vessels (marked by four white arrows) in the thermoacoustic images (figure 7.41(b)) is not as large as in the cross-sectional images (figure 7.41(b)), but the margins of the vessels were still clearly reconstructed.

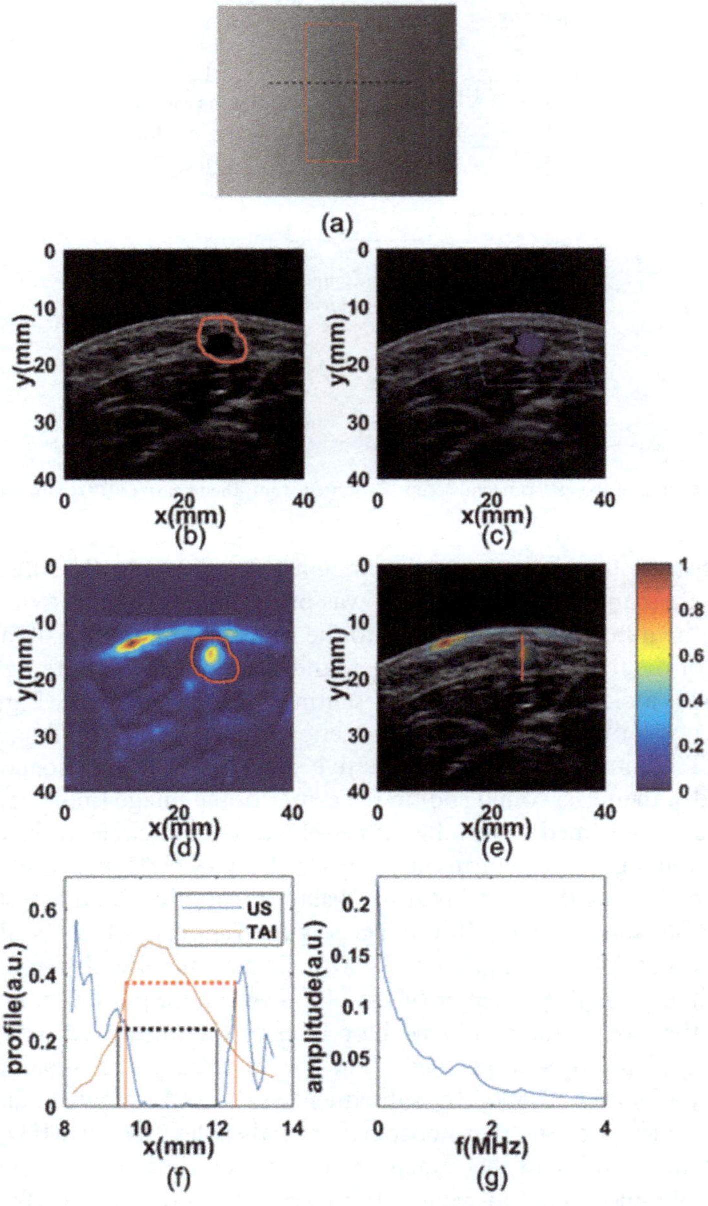

Figure 7.40. *In vivo* cross-sectional vascular imaging in the forearm. Photograph (a), ultrasound (b), color Doppler ultrasound (c), thermoacoustic (d), and overlaid (e) images. (f): The normalized TA and US profiles along a cut line (red) through the center of the blood vessel in (e). (g) The spectrogram of thermoacoustic signals. Color bar represents the relative TA signal. Reprinted from Zheng *et al* (2018), with the permission of AIP Publishing.

The lower contrast signal from the blood vessels seen in the sagittal plane (figure 7.41(b)) is largely related to the linear array transducer used and the cylindrical shape of the blood vessels and their orientation relative to the linear

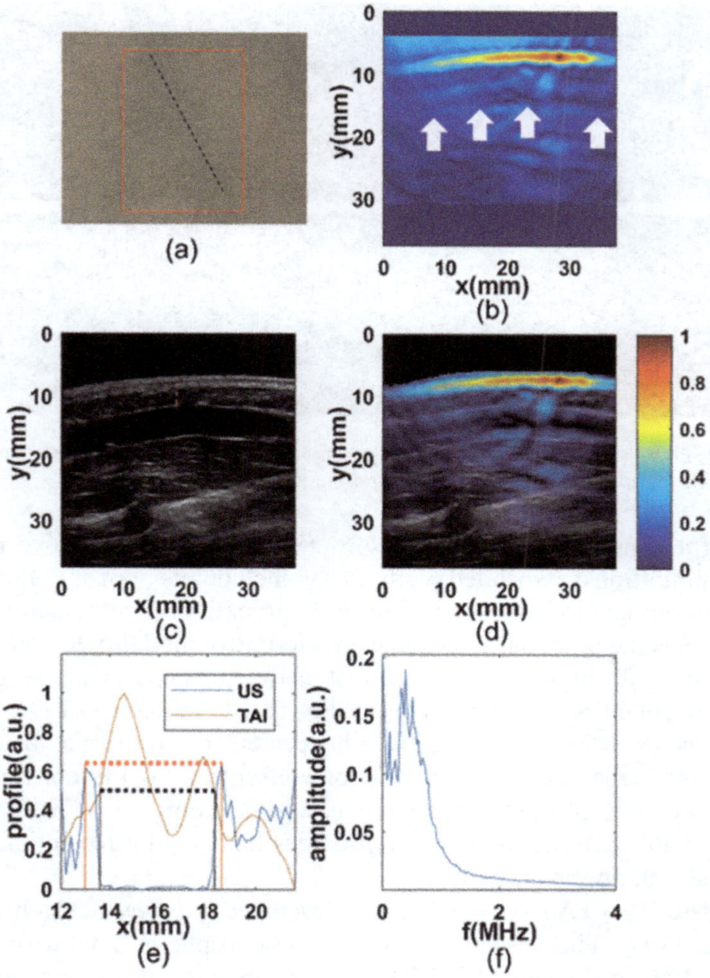

Figure 7.41. *In vivo* sagittal vascular imaging in the forearm. Photograph (a), thermoacoustic (b), ultrasound (c) and overlaid (d) images. (e): The normalized TA and US profiles along a cut line (red) through the center of the blood vessel in (d). (f) the spectrogram of thermoacoustic signals. Color bar represents the relative TA signal. Reprinted from Zheng *et al* (2018), with the permission of AIP Publishing.

array transducer. When a cylindrical target such as a blood vessel absorbs microwave energy, the resulting TA signals travel as a cylindrical wave. Therefore, most elements of the transducer can receive signals from one same target point in the cross section, while only a small portion of the elements (e.g. axial elements) can receive signals in the sagittal section.

7.6 Breast imaging

X-ray mammography is currently the most effective tool to detect breast cancer. However, the major limitation associated with x-ray is its low sensitivity for imaging dense breasts. For example, the sensitivity of x-ray for fat dominated breast tissue is

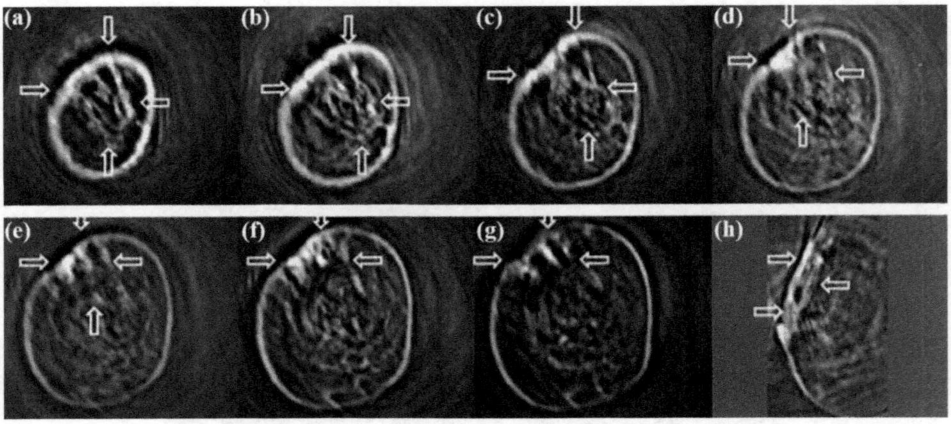

Figure 7.42. (a)–(g): Seven coronal TAT images. (h): one sagittal TAT image. The arrows indicate a large, lobulated enhancing mass. Reprinted with permission from Kruger *et al* (2000).

88%, while for dense breast tissue it is 62% (Sickles *et al* 2005, Boyd *et al* 1998). Additional limitations associated with x-ray include its ionizing radiation and considerable compression of breast during examination. Thermoacoustic tomography (TAT) has the potential to become an alternative modality for breast imaging primarily due to its high imaging contrast between a malignant lesion and the surrounding normal tissue, which can be as high as 6:1 (Joines *et al* 1994, Chaudhary *et al* 1984, Surowiec *et al* 1988). This enhancement of contrast is believed to be attributed to the higher water content and ion concentration of tumor tissue, leading to considerably increased tissue conductivity and dielectric constant for the tumor (Poplack *et al* 2004). In addition, TAT provides high spatial resolution, uses non-ionizing radiation, and is inexpensive.

Here we describe a TAT system that was developed to *in vivo* detect breast tumors (Kruger *et al* 1999). This system consisted of a hemispheric bowl with a radius of curvature of 175 mm where 64 1 MHz immersion transducers were arrayed in a spiral pattern spanning the surface of the hemisphere. The microwave source generated pulses of 1 ms width, 25 kW peak power at 433 MHz frequency, and the microwave was coupled to the breast via an 8 cm diameter, water-filled, cylindric waveguide. During the data collection, the patient lay prone and positioned one of her breasts through an aperture in the tabletop and immersed the breast in the imaging tank. The TA signals collected were first amplified by 66 dB and then digitized with 10 MHz sampling rate. The hemispheric bowl was mounted on a shaft that was rotated 32 times on its axis using a stepper motor. Thus, a total of 2048 samples were obtained for image reconstruction. The acquired TA signal was averaged 1024 times for each transducer.

A total of five patients with documented breast cancer were examined in this pilot study. We show TAT images for two of these patients. A series of seven coronal TAT images and one sagittal TAT image in the region of the cancerous mass for Patient #1 are shown in figure 7.42. The tumor was clearly identified (indicated by the arrows in figures 7.42(a)–(h)). Contrast increased approximately twofold in the region of this

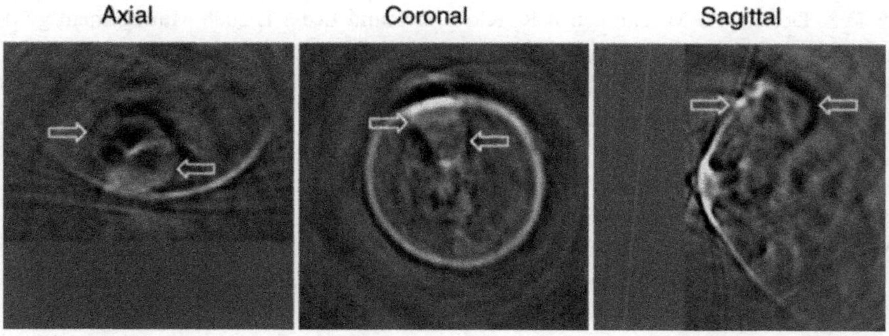

Figure 7.43. Three orthogonal views of TAT images showing an infiltrating ductal carcinoma (arrows). Reprinted with permission from Kruger *et al* (2000).

large mass. Patient #2 had a large palpable mass that was also clearly depicted by TAT. Three orthogonal TAT images (figure 7.43) show an area of contrast enhancement indicating a combination of postoperative changes and tumor.

References

Alamanos Y and Drosos A 2005 Epidemiology of adult rheumatoid arthritis *Autoimmun. Rev.* **4** 130–6

Altman R D 1990 Osteoarthritis differentiation from rheumatoid arthritis, causes of pain, treatment *Postgrad Med.* **87** 66–72

Balakrishnan L *et al* 2014 Differential proteomic analysis of synovial fluid from rheumatoid arthritis and osteoarthritis patients *Clinl. Proteom.* **11** 1–14

Bijlsma J W J, Berenbaum F and Lafeber F P J G 2011 Osteoarthritis: an update with relevance for clinical practice *Lancet* **377** 2115–26

Biswas S K, van Es P, Steenbergen W and Manohar S 2015 A method for delineation of bone surfaces in photoacoustic computed tomography of the finger *Ultrason. Imaging* **38** 63–76

Bolen J, Sniezek J, Thei K, Helmick C, Hootman J and Brady T 2005 Racial/ethnic differences in the prevalence and impact of doctor-diagnosed arthritis – United States 2002 *MMWR-Morbid Mortal. W.* **54** 119–23

Boyd N F, Lockwood G A and Byng J W *et al* 1998 Mammographic densities and breast cancer risk *Breast Dis.* **10** 113–26

Brown A K 2009 Using ultrasonography to facilitate best practice in diagnosis and management of RA *Nat. Rev. Rheumatol.* **5** 698–706

Chan W P, Lang P, Stevens M P, Sack K, Majumdar S, Stoller D W, Basch C and Genant H K 1991 Osteoarthritis of the knee: comparison of radiology, CT, and MR imaging to asses extent and severity *Am. J. Res.* **157** 799–806

Chaudhary S S, Mishra R K, Swarup A and Thomas J 1984 Dielectric properties of normal and malignant human breast tissues at radiowave and microwave frequencies *Indian J. Biochem. Biophys.* **21** 76–9

Chi Z, Zhao Y, Huang L, Zheng Z and Jiang H 2016 Thermoacoustic imaging of rabbit knee joints *Med. Phys.* **43** 6226–33

Chi Z, Zhao Y, Yang J, Li T, Zhang G and Jiang H 2019 Thermoacoustic tomography of *in vivo* human finger joints *IEEE T. on Biomed. Eng.* **66** 1598–608

Cooper D S, Doherty G M, Haugen B R, Kloos R T and Lee S L 2006 Management guidelines for patients with thyroid nodules and differentiated thyroid cancer *Thyroid* **16** 109–42

Delport H P 2015 Injuries of the knee *The Nuclear Medicine and Radiologic Imaging in Sports Injuries* ed A W J M Glaudemans, R A J O Dierckx, J L M A Gielen and J Zwerver (Berlin: Springer), pp 621–40

Deng Z and Li C 2016 Noninvasively measuring oxygen saturation of human finger-joint vessels by multi-transducer functional photoacoustic tomography *J. Biomed. Opt.* **21** 061009

Ding W, Ji Z, Ye F, Lou C and Xing D 2015 Near-field microwave distribution measurement with a point detector base on thermoacoustic effect *IEEE Trans. Microwave Theory Tech.* **63** 3272–6

Endo Y, Tezuka Y, Saito K and Ito K 2015 Dielectric properties and water contents of biological tissue after microwave heating *IEICE. Comex* **4** 231–2

Enewold L, Zhu K, Ron E, Marrogi A J, Stojadinovic A, Peoples G E and Devesa S S 2009 Rising thyroid cancer incidence in the United States by demographic and tumor characteristics, 1980–2005 *Cancer Epidemiol. Biomarkers Prev.* **18** 784–91

Erickson S J, Kneeland J B, Middleton W D, Jesmanowicz A, Hyde J, Lawson T L and Foley W D 1989 MR imaging of the finger: correlation with normal anatomic sections *Ajr. Am. J. Roentgenol.* **152** 1013–9

Firestein G S 2003 Evolving concepts of rheumatoid arthritis *Nature* **423** 356–61

Fu Y, Ji Z, Ding W, Ye F and Lou C 2014 Thermoacoustic imaging over large field of view for three-dimensional breast tumor localization: a phantom study *Med. Phys.* **41** 110701

Gabriel C, Gabriel S and Corthout E 1996a The dielectric properties of biological tissues: I. Literature survey *Phys. Med. Biol.* **41** 2231–49

Gabriel S, Lau R W and Gabriel C 1996b The dielectric properties of biological tissues: II. measurements in the frequency range 10 Hz to 20 GHz *Phys. Med. Biol.* **41** 2251–69

Gharib H, Papini E, Garber J R, Duick D S, Harrell R M, Hegedus L, Paschke R, Valcavi R and Vitti PAACE ACE AME Task Force on Thyroid Nodules 2016 American Association of Clinical Endocrinologists, American College of Endocrinology, and Associazione Medici Endocrinologi medical guidelines for clinical practice for the diagnosis and management of thyroid nodules–2016 update *Endocr. Pract.* **22** 622–39

Golnabi A H, Meany P M, Genimer S, Zhou T and Paulsen K D 2011 Microwave tomography for bone imaging *IEEE Int. Symp. on Biomedical Imaging: from Nano to Macro (Chicago, IL)* 956–9

Gupta P, Lenchik L, Wuertzer S D and Pacholke D A 2015 High-resolution 3-T MRI of the fingers: review of anatomy and common tendon and ligament injuries *AJR. Am. J. Roentgenol.* **204** 314–23

Guth S, Theune U, Aberle J, Galach A and Bamberger C M 2009 Very high prevalence of thyroid nodules detected by high frequency (13 MHz) ultrasound examination *Eur. J. Clin. Invest.* **39** 699–706

Hart D J and Spector T D 2000 Definition and epidemiology of osteoarthritis of the hand: a review *Osteoarthr. Cartilage* **8** s2–7

Hegedüs L 2004 The thyroid nodule *New Engl. J. Med.* **351** 1764–71

Hochberg M C 1991 Epidemiology of osteoarthritis: current concepts and new insights *J. Rheumatol. Suppl.* **27** 4–6

Hoelen C G A and de Mul F F M 2000 Image reconstruction for photo-acoustic scanning of tissue structures *Appl. Opt.* **39** 5872–83

Huang L, Yao L, Liu L, Rong J and Jiang H 2012 Quantitative thermoacoustic tomography: recovery of conductivity maps of heterogeneous media *Appl. Phys. Lett.* **101** 244106

Huang L, Li T and Jiang H 2017 Thermoacoustic imaging of hemorrhagic stroke: A feasibility study with a human skull *Med. Phys.* **44** 1494–9

Joines W T, Zhang Y, Li C and Jirtle R 1994 The measured electrical properties of normal and malignant human tissues from 50 to 900 MHz *Med. Phys.* **21** 547–50

Kruger R A, Miller K D, Reynolds H E, Kiser W L, Reinecke D R and Kruger G A 2000 Breast cancer in vivo: contrast enhancement with thermoacoustic CT at 434 MHz—feasibility study *Radiology* **216** 279–83

Kruger R A, Reinecke D R and Kruge G A 1999 Thermoacoustic computed tomography–technical considerations *Med. Phys.* **26** 1832–7

Lazebnik M, Converse M C, Booske J H and Hagness S C 2006 Ultrawideband temperature-dependent dielectric properties of animal liver tissue in the microwave frequency range *Phys. Med. Biol.* **51** 1941–55

Marrelli A, Cipriani P, Liakouli V, Carubbi F, Perricone C, Perricone R, Perricone R and Giacomelli R 2011 Angiogenesis in rheumatoid arthritis: a disease specific process or a common response to chronic inflammation *Autoimmun. Rev.* **10** 595–8

Mohajerani P, Koch M, Thürmel K, Haller B, Rummeny E J, Ntziachristos V and Meier R 2014 Fluorescence-aided tomographic imaging of synovitis in the human finger *Radiology* **272** 865–74

Nie L, Xing D, Zhou Q, Yang D and Guo H 2008 Microwave-induced thermoacoustic scanning CT for high-contrast and noninvasive breast cancer imaging *Med. Phys.* **35** 4026–32

Paessler H H and Mastrokalos D S 2003 Anterior cruciate ligament reconstruction using semitendinosus and gracilis tendons, bone patellar tendon, or quadriceps tendon–graft with press-fit fixation without hardware. A new and innovative procedure *Orthop. Clin. N. Am.* **34** 49–64

Plotkin B, Sampath S C, Sampath S C and Motamedi K 2016 MR imaging and US of the wrist tendons *Radiographics* **36** 1688–700

Poplack S P, Paulsen K and Hartov A *et al* 2004 Electromagnetic breast imaging: average tissue property values in women with negative clinical findings *Radiology* **231** 571–80

Rahib L, Smith B D, Aizenberg R, Rosenzweig A B, Fleshman J M and Matrisian L M 2014 Projecting cancer incidence and deaths to 2030: the unexpected burden of thyroid, liver, and pancreas cancers in the United States *Cancer Res.* **74** 2913

Reicher M A, Rauschning W, Gold R H, Bassett L W, Lufkin R B and Glenr W J 1985 High-resolution magnetic resonance imaging of the knee joint: normal anatomy *Am. J. Roentgenol.* **145** 895–902

Salvador S, Fear E, Okoniewski M and Matyas J 2009a Microwave imaging of the knee: on sensitivity, resolution and multiple tears detection *13th Int. Symp. on ANTEM/URSI (Toronto)* pp 1–4

Salvador S, Fear E, Okoniewski M and Matyas J 2009b Microwave imaging of the knee: application to ligaments and tendons *IEEE MTT-Int. Microwave Symp. on Digest (Boston, MA)* pp 1437–40

Sarzi-Puttini P, Cimmino M A, Scarpa R, Caporali R, Parazzini F, Zaninelli A, Atzeni F and Canesi B 2005 Osteoarthritis: an overview of the disease and its treatment strategies *Semin. Arthritis Rheu.* **35** 1–10

Sickles E A, Miglioretti D L and Ballard-Barbash R *et al* 2005 Performance benchmarks for diagnostic mammography *Radiology* **235** 775–90

Simon C J, Dupuy D E and Mayo-Smit W W 2005 Microwave ablation: principles and applications *Radiographics* **25** S69–83

Smith A and Moran C 2006 Soft tissue injuries of the knee *Surgery* **24** 376–81

Sun Y, Sobel E S and Jiang H 2011 First assessment of three-dimensional quantitative photoacoustic tomography for *in vivo* detection of osteoarthritis in the finger joint *Med. Phys.* **38** 4009–17

Surowiec A J, Stuchly S, Barr J and Swarup A 1988 Dielectric properties of breast carcinoma and the surrounding tissues *IEEE Trans. Biomed. Eng.* **35** 257–63

Van Es P, Biswas S K, Moens H, Steenbergen W and Manohar S 2015 Photoacoustic tomography of the human finger: towards the assessment of inflammatory joint diseases *SPIE Bios.* **9323** 611–22

Vasanth L C, Foo L F, Potter H G, Adler R S, Finzel K C, Pavlov H and Mandl L A 2010 Using magnetic resonance angiography to measure abnormal synovial blood vessels in early inflammatory arthritis: a new imaging biomarker *J. Rheumatol.* **37** 1129–35

Vecchia C L, Malvezzi M, Bosetti C, Garavello W, Bertuccio P, Levi F and Negri E 2015 Thyroid cancer mortality and incidence: a global overview *Int. J. Cancer* **136** 2187–95

Vogl T J, Nour-Eldin N A, Hammerstingl R M, Panahi B and Nnn N 2017 Microwave ablation (MWA): basics, technique and results in primary and metastatic liver neoplasms–review article *Fortschr. Röntgenstr.* **189** 1055–66

Vohra S, Arnold G, Doshi S and Marcantonio D 2011 Normal MR imaging anatomy of the knee *Magn. Reson. Imaging Clin. N. Am.* **19** 637–53

Wang X, Bauer D R, Russell W and Hao X 2012 Microwave-induced thermoacoustic imaging model for potential breast cancer detection *IEEE Trans. Biomed. Eng.* **59** 2782–91

Wang X, Huang L, Chi Z-H and Jiang H-B 2019 Microwave-induced thermoacoustic tomography for imaging human thyroid *Prog. Biochem. Biophys.* **46** 73

Wieschhoff G G, Sheehan S E, Wortman J R, Dyer G S M, Sodickson A D, Patel K I and Khurana B 2016 Traumatic finger injuries: what the orthopedic surgeon wants to know *RadioGraphics* **36** 1106–28

Wright A S, Sampson L A, Warner T F, Mahvi D M and Lee F T 2005 Radio frequency versus microwave ablation in a hepatic porcine model *Radiology* **236** 478–86

Xi L and Jiang H 2016 Integrated photoacoustic and diffuse optical tomography system for imaging of human finger joints *in vivo J. Biophotonics* **9** 213–7

Yao L, Gao G and Jiang H 2010 Quantitative microwave-induced thermoacoustic tomography *Med. Phys.* **37** 3752–9

Zhao Y, Chi Z, Huang L, Yang J and Jiang H 2017 Thermoacoustic tomography of *in vivo* rat brain *J. Innovative Opt. Health Sci.* **10** 1740001

Zhang S Y *et al* 2018 *Ex vivo* and *in vivo* monitoring and characterization of thermal lesions by high-intensity focused ultrasound and microwave ablation using ultrasonic Nakagami imaging *Int. J. Hyperthermia* **37** 1701–10

Zheng Z, Huang L and Jiang H 2018 Label-free thermoacoustic imaging of human blood vessels *in vivo Appl. Phys. Lett.* **113** 253702

Zhou T, Meaney P M, Pallone M J, Geimer S and Paulsen K D 2010 Microwave tomographic imaging for osteoporosis screening: a pilot clinical study *2010 Ann. Int. Conf. of the IEEE: EMBC (Buenos Aires)* 1218–21

Lightning Source UK Ltd.
Milton Keynes UK
UKHW050713270421
382700UK00003B/172